Self-Assessment Color Review of

Pediatric Emergency Medicine

Stephen Ludwig
MD, FAAP, FACEP
Professor of Pediatrics
The Children's Hospital of Philadelphia
and University of Pennsylvania School of Medicine
Philadelphia, Pennsylvania, USA

Patricia O. Brennan
FFAEM, FRCPCH
Consultant Pediatrician
Sheffield Children's Hospital, Sheffield, UK

Janet G. Yassa
FRCPCH, FFAEM, PhD
Consultant Pediatrician
Sheffield Children's Hospital, Sheffield, UK

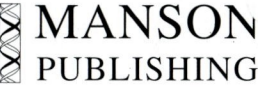
MANSON
PUBLISHING

Copyright © 2001 Manson Publishing Ltd
ISBN: 1–874545–46–4

A CIP catalogue record for this book is available from the British Library.

For full details of all Manson Publishing Ltd titles please write to:
Manson Publishing Ltd, 73 Corringham Road, London NW11 7DL, UK.

Commissioning editor: Jill Northcott
Project management: Paul Bennett
Copy-editing: Karen Bessant
Layout: Initial Typesetting Services
Cover design: Patrick Daly
Color reproduction: Tenon & Polert Colour Scanning Ltd, Hong Kong
Printed by: Grafos SA, Barcelona, Spain

Preface

Pediatric emergency medicine is becoming increasingly recognized as a subspecialty of both pediatrics and emergency medicine. There is little pictorial material on this subject which can be readily reviewed. This book aims to fill that gap.

This self-assessment book is designed to test the knowledge and skills of medical trainees and qualified practitioners managing children in the acute situation, whether they be working in general emergency medicine or primary care, or in the pediatric specialties of medicine, surgery, or orthopedics.

The book is designed to highlight the acute presentation and management of common and the not so common conditions in children. It covers the whole spectrum of pediatrics including medicine, surgery, orthopedics, ENT, ophthalmology, and dermatology. It emphasizes the differences between children and adults – 'children are not little adults.' There are differences in the significance of conditions in adults and children and in their assessment, investigation, and management.

This book is in the form of questions based on clinical cases each illustrated by photographs, X-rays, or investigations. The answers are given with discussion on various aspects of the case, for example, on differential diagnosis, complications, or management.

Stephen Ludwig
Patricia O. Brennan
Janet G. Yassa

Contributors

Elizabeth R. Alpern, MD
University of Pennsylvania School of
Medicine
The Children's Hospital of Philadelphia
Philadelphia, USA

Peter L. Barnett, MMBS, FRCAP,
MSc(epid), FACEM
Royal Children's Hospital
Parkville, Victoria, Australia

Michael J. Bell, FRCS
Children's Hospital
Western Bank, Sheffield, UK

Kathleen Berry, MD, FRCP(C), FFAEM
Birmingham Children's Hospital
Steelhouse Lane, Birmingham, UK

Patricia O. Brennan, FRCP, FFAEM,
FRCPCH
Children's Hospital
Western Bank, Sheffield, UK

Peter D. Bull, FRCS
Children's Hospital
Western Bank, Sheffield, UK

John Burke, FRCOphth
Royal Hallamshire Hospital
Glossop Road, Sheffield, UK

Jonathan Chan, FRCS, FRCOphth
Royal Hallamshire Hospital
Glossop Road, Sheffield, UK

Cindy Christian, MD
University of Pennsylvania School of
Medicine
The Children's Hospital of Philadelphia
Philadelphia, USA

Maureen Duggan, MD, FRCP,
FRCPCH, DTM&H
Mbarara University of Science and
Technology
Mbarara, Uganda

Joel Fein, MD
University of Pennsylvania School of
Medicine
The Children's Hospital of Philadelphia
Philadelphia, USA

Eric Freedlander, MD, FRCS (Plastic)Ed.
Children's Hospital
Western Bank, Sheffield, UK

Jane Lavelle, MD
University of Pennsylvania School of
Medicine
The Children's Hospital of Philadelphia
Philadelphia, USA

Stephen Ludwig, MD
University of Pennsylvania School of
Medicine
The Children's Hospital of Philadelphia
Philadelphia, USA

Ewen MacKinnon, MB, BS, FRCS,
FRCPCH
Children's Hospital
Western Bank, Sheffield, UK

Frank Oberklaid, MB, BS, MD, FRCAP,
DCH
Royal Children's Hospital
Melbourne, Australia

Betty L. Priestley, MB, FRCP, FRCPCH
Children's Hospital
Western Bank, Sheffield, UK

Robert Primak, MD, FRCP, FRCPCH
University of Sheffield
Children's Hospital
Western Bank, Sheffield, UK

Jenny Proimos, MB, BS, MPH, FRACP
Royal Children's Hospital
Parkville, Victoria, Australia

Brian I. Scott, FRCS (Orth)
Children's Hospital
Western Bank, Sheffield, UK

Alan Sprigg, DCH, DRCOG, DMRO,
FRCP(CH)
Children's Hospital
Western Bank, Sheffield, UK

G. Anthony Woodward, MD, MBA
Emergency Transport Service
Children's Hospital of Philadelphia
Philadelphia, USA

Janet G. Yassa, MBBS, DCH, DCP,
FRCPCH, FFAEM, PhD
Children's Hospital
Western Bank, Sheffield, UK

C.M. Yeoman, BDS, FDSRCS, PhD
Charles Clifford Dental Hospital
Sheffield, UK

Broad classification of cases

Abbreviations

ABC airways, breathing, and circulation

AIDS acquired immunodeficiency syndrome

ASO antistreptococcal

APLS advanced pediatric life support

ATLS advanced trauma life support

BCG bacillus Calmette–Guérin

CNS central nervous system

CSF cerebrospinal fluid

CT computed tomography

DNA deoxyribonucleic acid

ECG electrocardiogram

EEG electroencephalogram

ENT ear, nose, and throat

ESR erythrocyte sedimentation rate

FEV_1 forced expiratory volume in 1 second

FVC forced expiratory vital capacity

HBsAg hepatitis B surface antigen

HIV human immunodeficiency virus

HLA human leukocyte antigen

$PaCO_2$ arterial carbon dioxide

PCV packed cell volume

RNA ribonucleic acid

1 A 12-year-old girl fell out of a tree onto some metal railings which pierced her thigh. Emergency services cut the railings and brought her to the emergency department (1). What should the first actions of the emergency receiving team include?

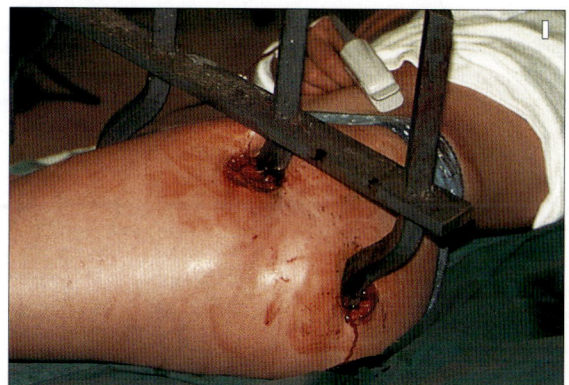

2 This 8-year-old child was beaten by her parent for misbehaving in school (2). What condition might you anticipate? How should you make the diagnosis?

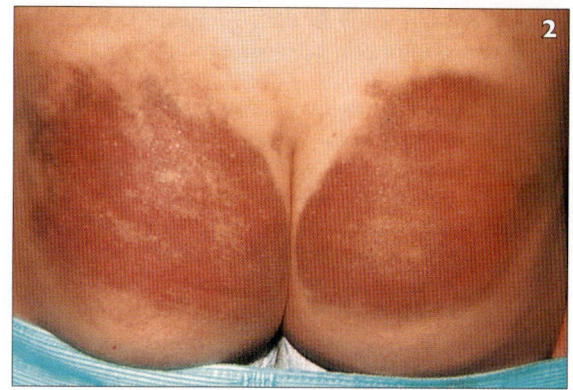

3 This young boy has a vesicular lesion above and below his right eye (3).
i. What is the next important step in his examination?
ii. What tissue layers of the eye can be affected in this infection?

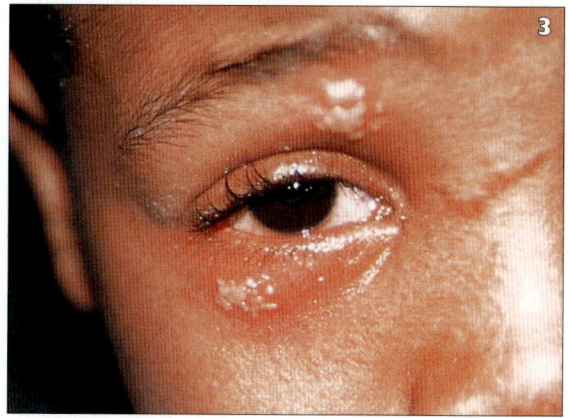

1 Although this girl's leg injuries look and are severe, they are not actually life threatening. Their evaluation is, therefore, carried out during the secondary survey and their treatment commenced during the definitive care phase.

Initially the primary survey must be carried out in the familiar pattern of:

A Airway and cervical spine management.
B Breathing.
C Circulation and hemorrhage control.
D Disability.
E Exposure.

Life threatening problems found during this survey must be treated as they are identified.

In this girl, her airway and breathing were uncompromized. Intravenous access was secured, however, as hypovolemic shock would be a danger. It is difficult to estimate the blood loss from the time of the accident to the arrival at the hospital. Pain control is also necessary early in the treatment. The railings were later removed and wound toilet carried out in the operating room.

2 This severe beating may result in rhabdomyolysis and myoglobinuria that may in turn lead to acute renal failure. To make the diagnosis check the child's urine – if a test strip is positive for hem and the urinalysis does not show red blood cells, then you can assume it is a false positive caused by myoglobin. A serum creatine phosphokinase will also document massive tissue destruction. The child should be admitted to hospital to ensure good fluid intake and urine output.

This is a severe injury and must be reported as a case of child abuse. The intention of the parents appears to have been to chastise the child to teach her the importance of attending school. However, the severity of the punishment is unacceptable and the child must be kept in a safe place until a multiagency child protection investigation is undertaken.

3 i. The next step in the examination would be to stain the conjunctiva and cornea with fluoroscein. The lesion seen was consistent with corneal dendritic ulcer. This is diagnostic of herpes simplex infection and the patient requires referral to an ophthalmic surgeon.

ii. Herpes simplex can affect the superficial epithelial layers of the cornea and conjunctiva. However, it can also give a spectrum of eye disease affecting the stromal layers. This can result in stromal keratitis, stromal opacities, corneal vascularization, and perforations. Intraocular involvement causes uveitis. In developed countries herpes simplex is the commonest cause of corneal blindness and it is particularly troublesome in neonates and patients with immune problems, e.g. AIDS and transplant patients.

4 This child presented to the emergency department with a mass in the midline of his neck (4).

i. What simple test will help you to determine the origin of the mass?

ii. Why should this condition occur in a school age child?

iii. What is your differential diagnosis?

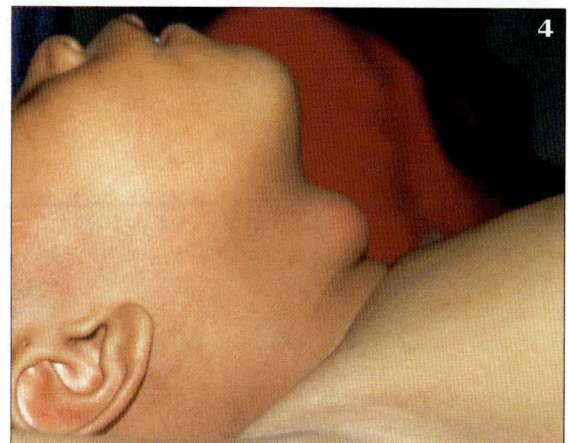

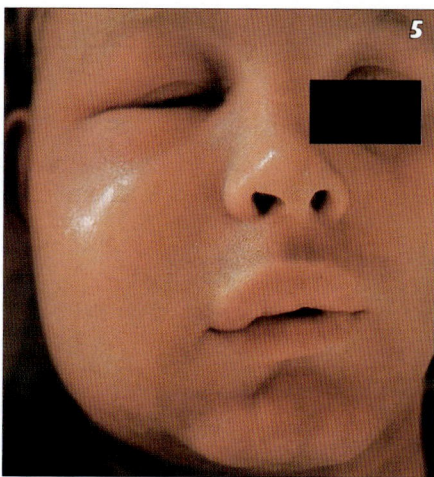

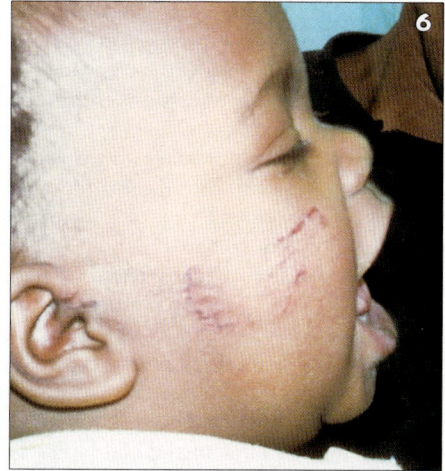

5 This patient developed a right-sided facial swelling 2 days after experiencing intermittent pain in the ipsilateral maxilla (5).

i. What is the probable cause of the swelling?

ii. Discuss the management.

iii. If untreated what severe complications may result?

6 This 8-month-old girl was presented to the emergency department with marks on her face (6). She had been left with her older siblings (ages 2 and 5 years), in the care of her father. The mother returned to find marks on the infant's cheek. What is the mark and how would you go about evaluating it?

4 i. This child has a thyroglossal duct cyst, which lies between the hyoid bone and the suprasternal notch. It is a midline structure that results from the persistence of the thyroglossal duct remnant. If you ask the child to put out his tongue or to swallow, the cyst will move upwards.
ii. Although the thyroglossal duct remnant may have been present since birth, it may go undetected until an infection causes it to enlarge and fill with fluid. Treatment of this condition includes initial antibiotic therapy to eradicate the infection and subsequent surgical removal of the cyst and remnant.
iii. The differential diagnosis includes: an inflamed lymph node, a branchial cleft cyst, a cystic hygroma, a ranula, and a sternomastoid muscle hematoma.

5 i. The patient has a spreading cellulitis associated with an acute abscess from a maxillary tooth. This could spread to deeper tissues such as the infraorbital facial soft tissue planes or the submandibular region. Trauma or caries in a tooth predisposes to an abscess usually caused by a staphylococcal or streptococcal organism. In primary dentition the acute abscess is usually superficial.
ii. Removal of the tooth and, if indicated, intraoral drainage in the upper buccal sulcus is urgently required. Suitable broad spectrum antibiotic therapy to control the further spread of infection is also necessary. Assess the remaining dentition. If dental neglect was the cause prophylactic advice to the parents about routine dental care is also needed to prevent further episodes.
iii. If untreated cavernous sinus thrombosis is a possible severe complication.

6 This is a human bite mark to the face. The mark consists of abrasions in an almost circular distribution. Bites are common pediatric injuries and can occur during fights, play, sports, sexual activity, or maltreatment.
  Human bites result in crushing of the skin and abrasions and are distinguished from animal bites by their pattern (circular, oval, parentheses). A central suck mark is occasionally seen. The intercanine distance can help to determine whether the bite is from an adult or a child. The adult arch is generally 2.5–4.0 cm (1–1.5 in) in diameter, although there is overlap between the size of the adult and child's dental arch.
  If there is concern about child maltreatment, additional steps may assist in determining the biter of the child. The bite mark can be swabbed and the swab sent for salivary analysis of ABO grouping. Photographic evidence can also be compared with dental moulds of suspected perpetrators (although this is rarely done). A skeletal survey may reveal occult fractures.
  This infant had been bitten by her older sibling.

7 This boy shows marked facial swelling (7).
i. What is the cause?
ii. How soon after the injury can this degree of swelling be expected?
iii. What immediate clinical steps must be taken in the examination of a child admitted with these signs in the head and neck?

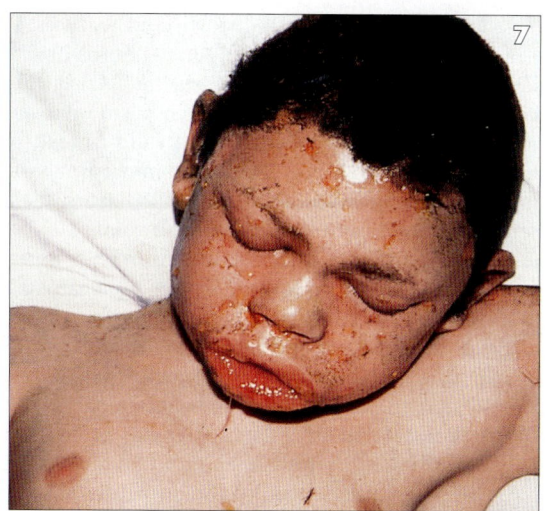

8 An adolescent boy struck another child in the jaw. He now complains of pain at the ulnar aspect of his left hand. There is swelling on inspection and tenderness on palpation. This X-ray of his left hand was taken (8).
i. What is the diagnosis?
ii. What would determine optimal treatment?
iii. What complication should be looked for?

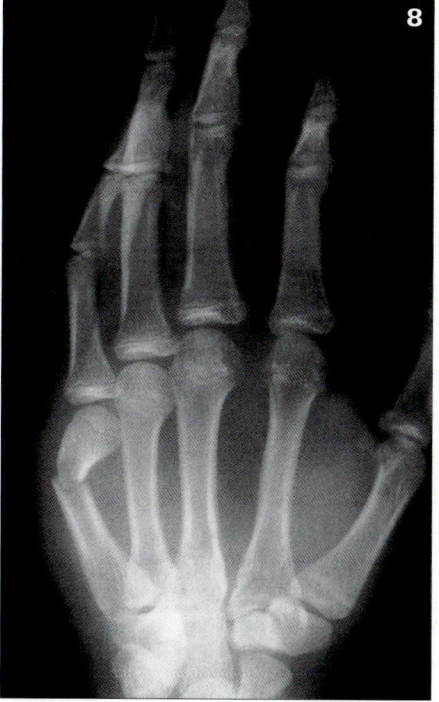

7 i. The gross edema with distortion of features, swelling of eyelids, lips and ears has been caused by flash burns. Any facial burns or scalding can result in this appearance.
ii. Significant swelling is seen within 24 hours of injury and the patient must be warned to expect it. The main mechanism involved is increased capillary permeability to both water and protein causing fluid to leak out into the extravascular compartment. Histamine release from heat injured mast cells is the most likely cause of the increased permeability, but other mediators such as prostaglandins, thromboxane, serotonin, and kinins may also play a role.
iii. The immediate medical treatment must ensure that an adequate airway is secured and any signs of respiratory difficulty (wheeze, stridor, hoarseness, and use of secondary muscles of respiration) identified. In flame burns, carbon particles may be present in the nose or mouth, and there may be evidence of singeing of nasal hairs.

The history will make clear the etiology of the injury. Burns in an enclosed space should alert to the possibility of inhalational injury. The airways can be compromized by extrinsic edema or intrinsic damage to the mucosal lining of the bronchial tree. Urgent endotracheal intubation should be considered and expert advice obtained.

Depending on the cause of the burn, the possibility of damage to the eyes must be considered. The globes should be examined before developing edema closes the eyelids. Saline irrigation should be used and antibiotic drops instilled. If there is any doubt, an ophthalmologist should be consulted.

It is important to anticipate that swelling will supervene within hours of injury. For this reason, even patients with no signs require admission and observation until the time span for development of edema has passed.

8 i. This fracture is called a 'boxer's fracture' because it is usually caused by throwing a punch. The fifth metacarpal is the most commonly fractured bone of the hand. On examination there is swelling, tenderness, and decreased prominence of the affected knuckle with finger flexion.
ii. The presence or absence of rotational displacement determines the treatment options. This can be assessed by noting the lack of parallel alignment of the nail beds in extension or digit overlap in flexion. Isolated shaft fractures usually have minimal displacement and may be treated with closed reduction and immobilization. Neck fractures usually have palmar displacement and should be treated with closed reduction. Early immobilization by neighbour strapping to the ring finger limits the degree of extension following the injury. Intra-articular fractures require open reduction and fixation to restore the joint surface. Importantly, any residual rotational malalignment will result in functional impairment.
iii. Punches to the mouth frequently involve a puncture wound by human teeth. The fist must be carefully checked as any wound will be grossly contaminated with mouth flora.

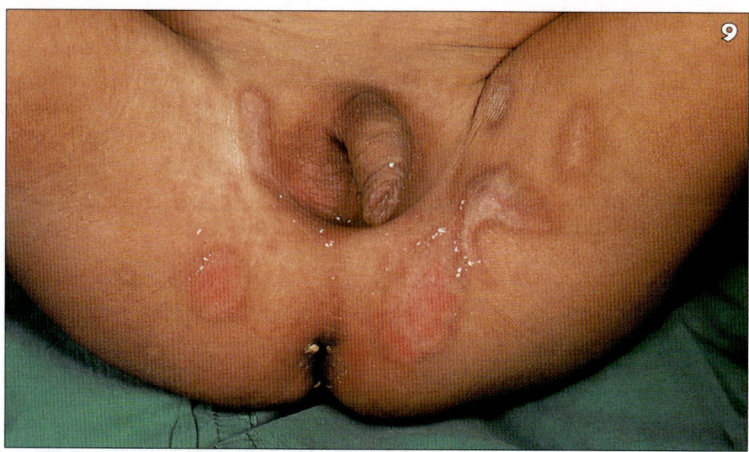

9 A small boy presented with a 2 cm (0.75 in) circular ulcerated lesion to his forearm. On further examination he was found to have the healed diaper (nappy) rash shown (**9**). Describe the nature of the diaper rash and discuss its possible causes.

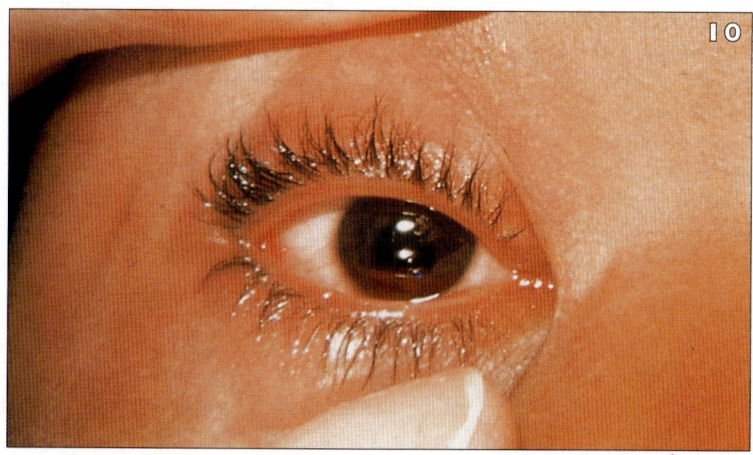

10 An 8-year-old boy was hit in the eye with a ball. What is the significance of the finding shown (**10**)?

9 Young children in diapers occasionally develop a rash in the diaper area. This appears to be less common in developed countries since the widespread use of disposable diapers.

The commonest causes of diaper rash include conditions where chronic irritation takes place, e.g. poor hygiene with ammoniacal irritation and sensitivity to washing powder or fabric softener. Other common causes include monilial infection, seborrheic dermatitis spreading from the creases and associated with cradle cap, and psoriasis. Rarely conditions such as Hans–Schuller–Christian disease can present with a rash in the diaper area. A good history and a good general examination must therefore be undertaken on all children with this common presentation.

Management of the condition involves good hygiene, barrier creams, and treatment of both the primary condition and any secondary infection.

The rash in this case appears to have consisted of four discrete circumscribed areas, not consistent with any of the causes above. The nature of the healed lesions suggests that the rash consisted of ulcerated areas. He also had an ulcer of the arm. On further questioning the parents said that the boy had a similar eruption on his forehead, nose and cheeks 6 months previously and had a spiral fracture of his femur 3 months previously. The spectrum and nature of the injuries caused a child protection investigation to be initiated. The diaper rash, ulcer of the arm, and facial rash were subsequently proved to have been caused by the application of a caustic substance.

10 He has a hyphema or bleed into the anterior chamber of the eye. This requires urgent ophthalmological referral.

Corneal staining following a hyphema results in decreased visual acuity and occasionally even amblyopia. Predictors for corneal staining are duration of hyphema, raised intraocular pressure, the presence of corneal damage, and rebleeding during the recovery period. The latter is a particularly bad prognostic sign and analgesics which alter hemostasis such as aspirin are contraindicated. (Aspirin would be contra-indicated as an analgesic anyway in a child of this age in view of the risk of Reye's syndrome.)

11 A 7-year-old girl reports a minor head injury 2 days before presentation. She presents now with a markedly swollen scalp and upper face. She is in no respiratory distress.

i. What does the CT scan show (**11**)?

ii. What is the treatment?

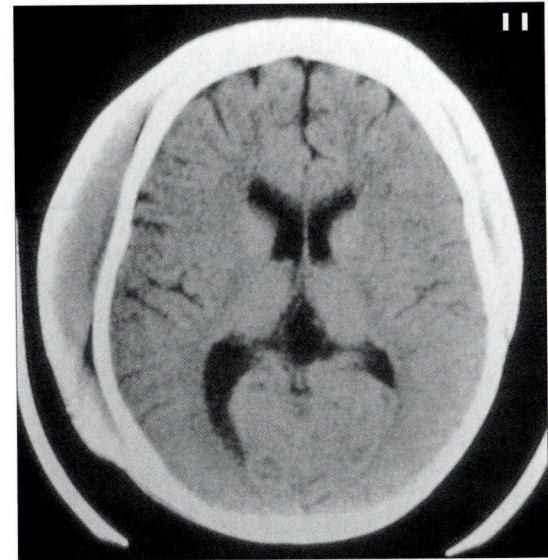

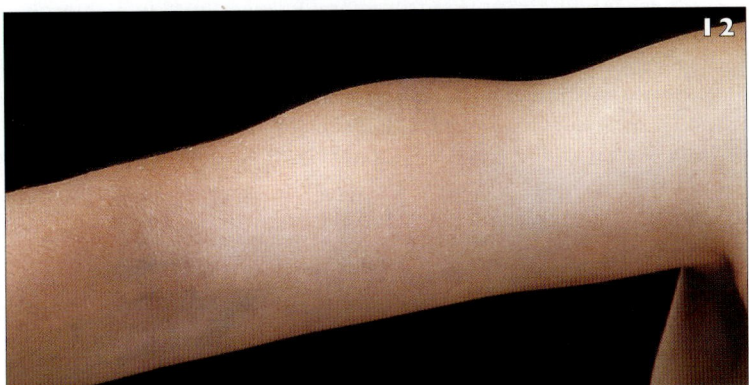

12 A 10-year-old child with insulin-dependent diabetes mellitus was staying for the weekend with her friend. In the previous 24 hours she felt ill, was off her food, appeared hot, and vomited. In the last 2 hours she became drowsy. It was not certain whether she had taken her regular injections and she seemed to have become worse. Her friend's mother brought her to the emergency department.

i. What is the sign shown (**12**), and how is it caused?

ii. What is the underlying diagnosis?

iii. What would be the principles of your management?

11 i. There is no evidence of intracranial injury or cranial fracture. The CT scan does demonstrate bilateral subgaleal bleeding. This occurs between the periosteum and the epicranial aponeurosis. It is usually firm and fluctuant and it crosses the suture lines. It can be associated with symptoms of acute blood loss and is sometimes seen in infants following a traumatic delivery.

ii. As always ensure adequate ABC. Consider evaluation of prothrombin and partial thromboplastin time to look for underlying reasons for excessive subgaleal blood with a minor closed head injury. The hematoma itself rarely requires treatment.

12 i. The sign is lipomatosis due to fat deposition which is caused by injecting insulin repeatedly at the same site rather than rotating the sites.

ii. She appears to have developed ketoacidosis which was probably precipitated by an infection and possibly missing an insulin injection.

iii. This is a life-threatening medical emergency and the following steps are required and should be accurately recorded:

- Assessment of her general condition applying the ABC resuscitation principles.
- Assessment of her hydration. Five per cent dehydration would show dry mucous membranes and loss of skin turgor. Ten per cent dehydration gives sunken eyes and poor capillary return while over 10% dehydration gives a poor pulse and low blood pressure with acidotic respiration and abdominal pain. Intravenous 0.9% saline should be started to begin correction of the dehydration carefully. Too rapid or excessive rehydration may lead to cerebral edema. Potassium chloride must be added to the fluids to correct body deficits.
- Further investigations should be undertaken including: weight, blood glucose, urea and electrolytes, bicarbonate, full blood count, PCV, disseminated intravascular coagulation screen and blood culture, and urine for ketones and culture.
- Intravenous soluble insulin infusion is commenced via a separate infusion pump at the rate of 0.1 U/kg bodyweight per hour.
- Intravenous bicarbonate is only considered if the child's pH <7 and the child is in circulatory failure.
- Admission and further management.

13 This child presented with a history of pallor, sweating, tremor, abdominal pain, and irritability (**13**). She has been attending the hospital for relapsing nephrotic syndrome.

i. What simple test would you do to explain the signs and symptoms?

ii. What is the role of the emergency department doctor in managing such children?

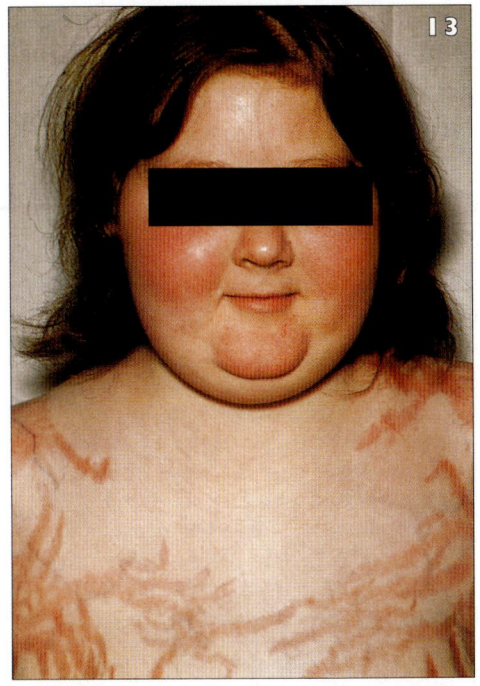

14 This girl recently had the upper part of her ear pierced to wear an ear stud (**14**). What complication has ensued?

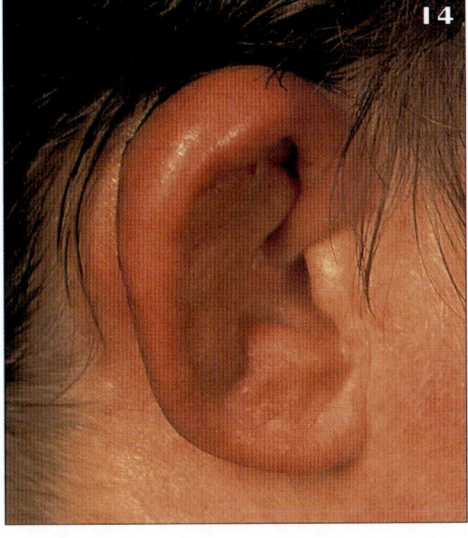

13 i. The child has Cushingoid features caused by repeated treatment with high dose corticosteroids given for her relapsing nephrotic syndrome. This has lead to suppression of her adrenal gland resulting in hypoglycemia.

Hypoglycemia causes sympathetic nerve stimulation leading to tachycardia, palpitation, pallor, perspiration, and tremor. It can also cause CNS dysfunction such as ataxia, mood changes, confusion, convulsions, coma, and general symptoms such as abdominal pain and headaches. This child needs to be assessed for both steroid toxicity and adrenal suppression.

A finger-prick test for blood glucose in the emergency department would reveal hypoglycemia (a plasma glucose of <2.6 mmol/l [<46.8 mg/dl] in the older infant and child).

Other causes of hypoglycemia include:

- Stress from prolonged fasting and high metabolic demand as in infection with fever.
- Poorly controlled insulin-dependent diabetes mellitus.
- Ketotic hypoglycemia in a thin child with inadequate glycogen stores and ineffective gluconeogenesis after poor food intake.
- Hormonal causes such as primary adrenal insufficiency and hypopituitarism and hyperinsulinism caused by neisidioblastosis.
- Inherited primary enzyme deficiencies affecting carbohydrate metabolism such as galactosemia, fat metabolism such as medium chain acyl-co-A dehydrogenase deficiency or aminoacid metabolism such as methyl-malonic aciduria.

ii. The role of the emergency department doctor in the management of hypoglycemic patients involves three aspects:

- Collection of specimens including blood for blood glucose, lactate, alanine, free fatty acids, ß-hydroxybutyrate, carnitine, cortisol, insulin and growth hormone, and urine for organic acids and acyl-carnitines.
- Correction of the hypoglycemia by giving milk by mouth if the child is fit enough. Otherwise give intravenous 10% glucose, 0.7 ml/kg/min for 3 minutes then continue with 10% dextrose infusion at a rate of 0.1 ml/kg/min. Check the blood glucose at 5 minute intervals until the blood glucose rises to 5–8 mmol/l (90–144 mg/dl). Glucagon 1 mg intramuscularly may be tried if intravenous access is difficult, but is only effective if there are enough glycogen stores in the liver.
- Correction of any other deficit, e.g. hydrocortisone intravenously if hypopituitarism is suspected.

14 This girl has severe perichondritis and cellulitis of the right pinna. Admission for intravenous antibiotic therapy is required. The offending ear stud should be removed. There may ultimately be a poor cosmetic result as a consequence of the perichondritis and cartilage damage.

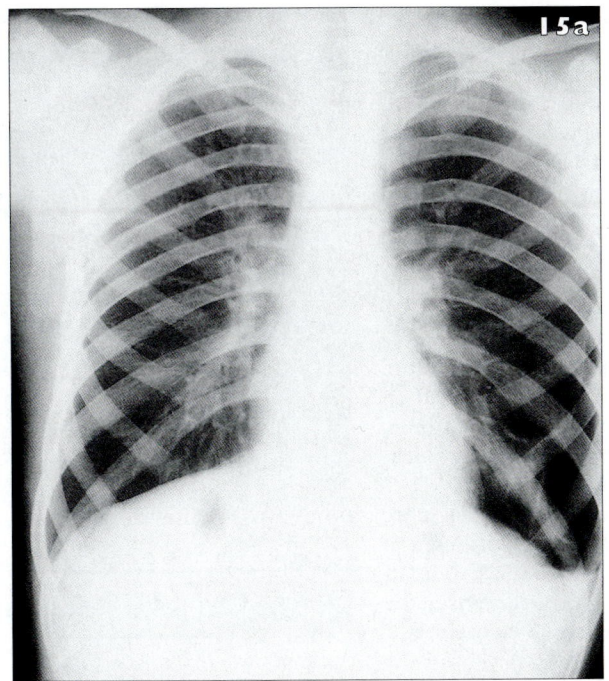

15 An 11-year-old boy presented with sudden onset of left-sided chest pain and shortness of breath.
i. What do you see on the chest X-ray (**15a**)?
ii. How would you manage this child?

16 A 3-week-old infant presented acutely with the ocular findings shown (**16**).
i. What is the differential diagnosis?
ii. What tests might you consider?

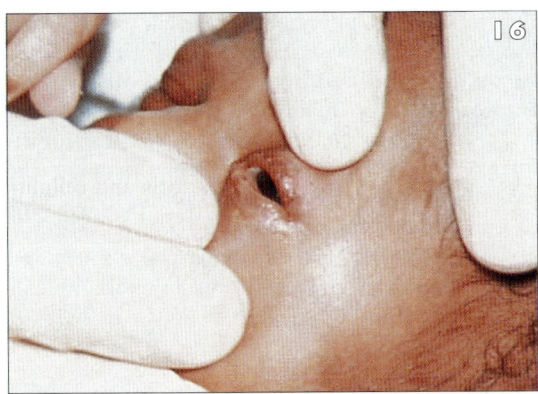

15 i. There is a shallow, left-sided pneumothorax. The mediastinum is central. The lung edge can be seen (small arrowheads, **15b**) and a horizontal fluid level is seen on this erect film at the left base (large arrowhead, **15b**). This horizontal line on an erect chest film separates air (pneumothorax) from the fluid (containing protein or blood). Fluid levels are visible only on an erect film.

Spontaneous pneumothorax is uncommon in childhood. It more commonly occurs as a complication of other conditions such as asthma, bronchiolitis, staphylococcal pneumonia, and trauma.

ii. If the oxygen saturation is more than 95% in air, after settling and reassuring the child, no active treatment is required. Otherwise, the pneumothorax should be drained.

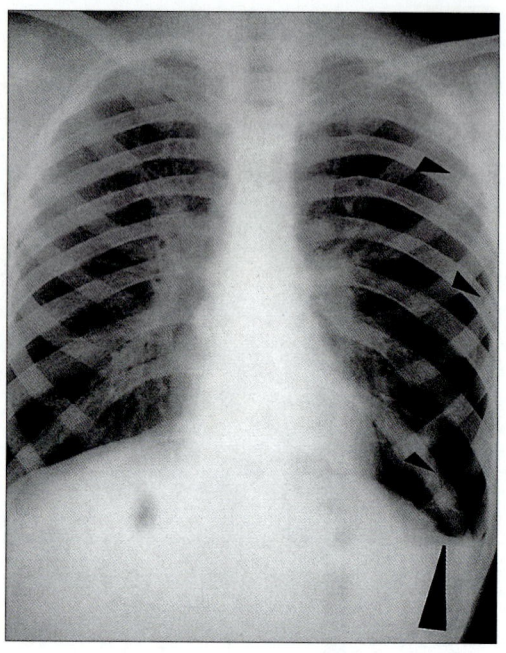

16 i. The child has signs of conjuctivitis. Many cases of neonatal conjunctivitis are caused by organisms acquired during vaginal delivery making *Neisseria gonorrhoea* and *Chlamydia trachomatis* important etiologies. However, chemicals, other bacteria, and viruses can also cause the disease. *Haemophilus influenzae* and *Streptococcus pneumoniae, Escherichia coli,* and other pathogens can cause conjunctivitis in early infancy as well as in older children. These pathogens may be transmitted either from the baby's own nasopharyngeal passages or from those of the carers.

ii. Physical examination alone is inadequate for diagnosis. A Gram stain looking for the presence of polymorphonuclear cells as well as Gram-negative intracellular diplococci aids in management. Culture of eye swabs for *N. gonorrhoea* and nasopharyngeal culture for *C. trachomatis* should be considered in all patients. Serologic tests for chlamydia on conjunctival secretions would give an early diagnosis.

This child was admitted and treated for suspected gonococcal conjunctivitis with an intravenous third generation cephalosporin and eye irrigation. If this child had gonnorrhea and was not treated promptly, he may have developed the complications of gonnorrheal conjunctivitis of corneal ulceration and perforation. Cultures were positive for chlamydia. The baby was subsequently treated with a 3 week course of oral erythromycin and erythromycin ophthalmic ointment.

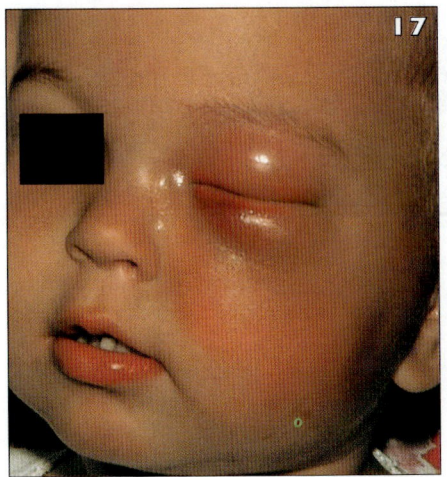

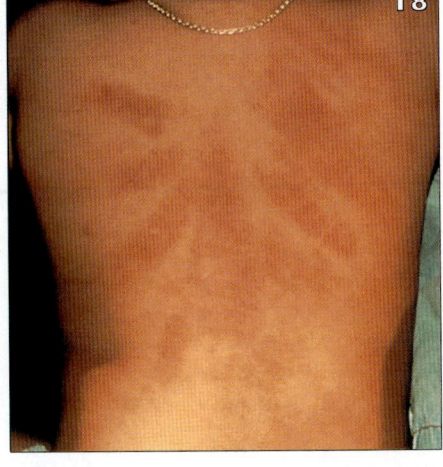

17 This 15-month-old child presented with a 24 hour history of fever and increasing swelling and redness of the periorbital region (**17**).
i. What is the diagnosis?
ii. What is the likely infecting organism and what may be the source of the infection?
iii. How should the child be managed?

18 A boy was brought to the emergency department for evaluation of a fever and during the examination these findings were noticed (**18**).
i. What is the most likely cause of the lesions on his back?
ii. Would this be considered child abuse?

19 A patient had a ventricular peritoneal shunt in place. He had signs of increasing intracranial pressure for 2–3 days before admission (lethargy, vomiting, and headache) and deteriorated to a near arrest. He was intubated and developed unilateral chest sounds with asymmetrical chest expansion.
i. What does the X-ray show (**19**)?
ii. What is the therapy?
iii. What are the possible reasons for increased intracranial pressure in this child?

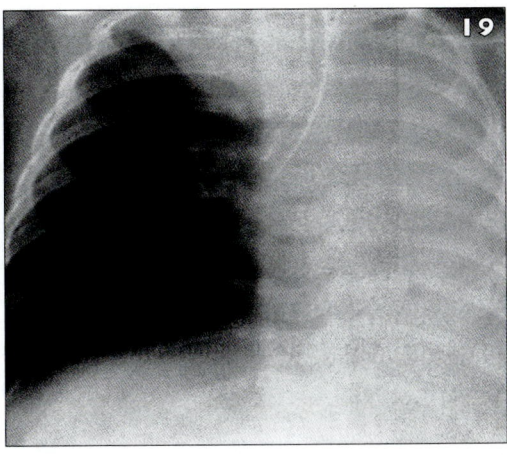

17 i. This child has redness and congestion of the eyelids, orbital tissues, and bulbar conjunctiva. The diagnosis is periorbital cellulitis.

ii. If there is no history of local trauma or skin lesion, the most likely organism in young children is *Haemophilus influenzae* type B (characterized by magenta discoloration of the skin of the eyelids, as in this child), followed by *Streptococcus pneumoniae*.

The likely causative organisms change with the age of the child. *Staphylococcus aureus* and Gram-negative bacilli are more common in babies and *S. aureus* infection after trauma to the skin in older children.

The infection may spread from an ethmoid sinusitis in infants or from the maxillary and frontal sinuses in older children. Complications include cavernous sinus thrombosis and meningitis.

iii. This child needs to be admitted to hospital and given intravenous antibiotics. Improvement would be expected within 48–72 hours. Lack of improvement suggests that surgical drainage is needed.

18 i. These lesions are most likely caused by 'coining', a culturally-based effort to heal a person's illness by rubbing hot coins along his skin.

ii. Most clinicians feel that the practice is relatively benign, but provides little medical help to the patient. There is a difference between childhood injuries caused by culturally based therapies and those considered child abuse. It is important to take into consideration the intent of the perpetrator when deciding to report a finding as suspicious for child abuse. However, most Western societies would consider a traditional remedy which was painful and caused injuries and which had no therapeutic basis unacceptable within their society. It should therefore be discouraged and the aim should be to stop it by education rather than by the child protection process.

19 i. The chest X-ray shows atelectasis (white out) of the left lung with the endotracheal tube in the right main bronchus. This should not be mistaken for a pneumothorax involving the hyperinflated right lung.

ii. Therapy involves correct positioning of the endotracheal tube and eventual re-expansion of the affected lung. There is no reason to place a needle or chest tube as this could lead to serious compromise in the patient.

iii. The intracranial pressure could have been the result of: blockage of the shunt, usually at the ventricular or peritoneal end, disconnection or breakage of the tubing of the shunt, and an overactive shunt, leading to collapse of the ventricle and interference with drainage.

20 A boy had a swelling over his sternum on getting up one morning and developed parotid swellings over the next 24 hours. What is the swelling shown (20), and what is the underlying condition? What other complications of this condition do you know?

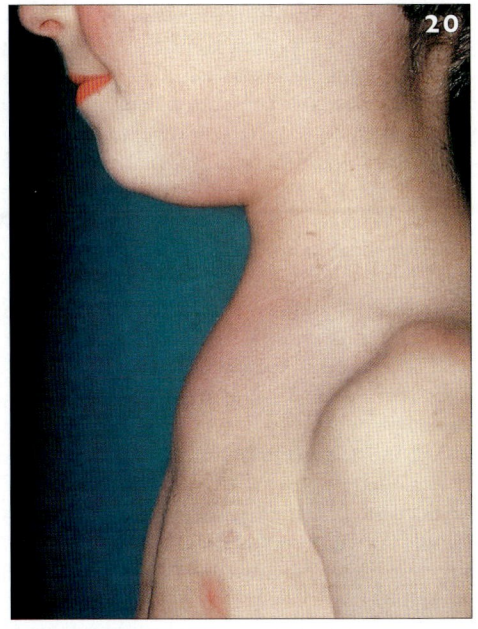

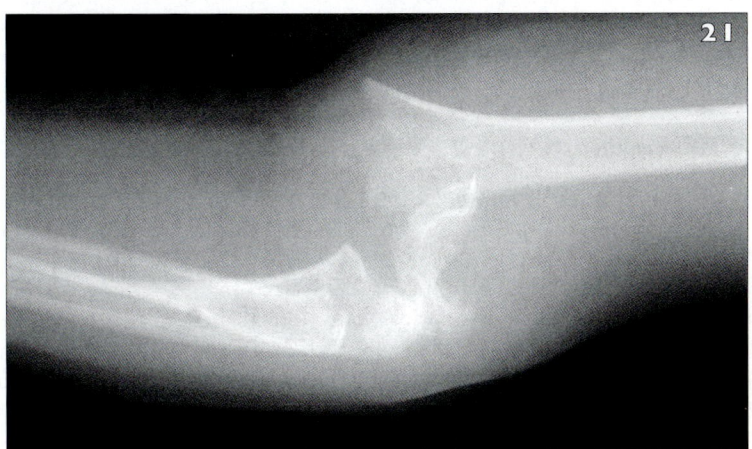

21 i. From the evidence in the X-ray shown (21), what is the diagnosis in this child?
ii. What clinical features must be sought and documented? What are the important complications of this injury?

20 He has a condition known as presternal myxedema associated with a mumps parotitis. It is a pitting edema over the sternum thought to be caused by blockage of the local lymphatic vessels.

Mumps usually presents as a nonsuppurative enlargement of the parotid glands in children of 5–15 years. However, approximately 30% of cases are thought to be subclinical and others can present with one of the many complications. These include: aseptic meningitis, orchitis, pancreatitis, mastitis, myocarditis, hepatitis, thyroiditis, and thrombocytopenic purpura. An infection with mumps virus is also thought to be an etiological factor in some cases of diabetes mellitus.

21 i. This is a grossly displaced supracondylar humeral fracture which is particularly common in children.

ii. The degree of displacement indicates this was a relatively high energy injury and thus soft tissue damage at the elbow should be assessed before management of the bone injury begins.

The most important complication is occlusion or laceration of the brachial artery as it is pulled backwards over the sharp fracture edge of the proximal fragment. An assessment of capillary circulation in the hand and the presence of the radial pulse should always be sought and documented. Diminished distal perfusion mandates urgent orthopedic advice on whether emergency reduction to restore distal circulation is required.

A long term complication resulting from prolonged ischemia (more than 4–6 hours) is a compartment syndrome which results in rapid muscle death. Late muscle fibrosis causes the functionless and untreatable clawed hand of Volkmann's ischemic contracture. The rapid onset of a large and tense swelling may further compromise distal circulation and in addition makes closed reduction difficult. Even with normal distal circulation some would argue that the swelling which should be anticipated with this sort of injury makes emergency reduction necessary.

It is important to recognize that ischemia of the forearm musculature can occur because of diminished perfusion through the anterior interosseous branch of the brachial artery even though the radial branch may retain a palpable pulse. For this reason when assessing the patient for development of a compartment syndrome the cardinal features should be regarded as: increasing and severe forearm pain exacerbated by passive extension of the fingers, clinically obvious tension in the muscle compartment, and evidence of diminished distal circulation.

Other complications include neuropraxia of the median, radial and ulnar nerves resulting from stretching at the time of injury. The sensory status of the arm should be recorded. These 'nerve lesions in continuity' recover spontaneously over months.

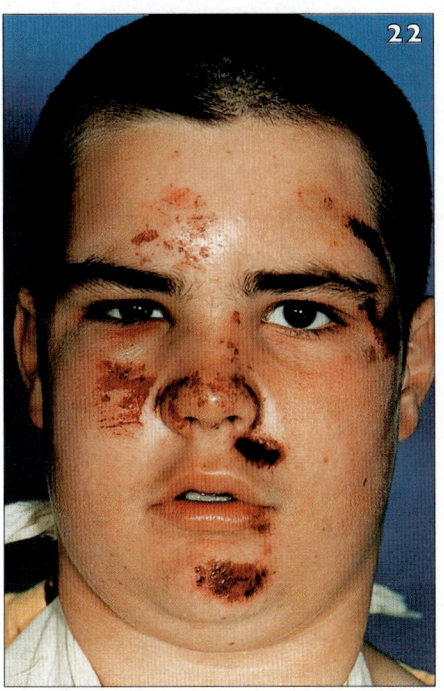

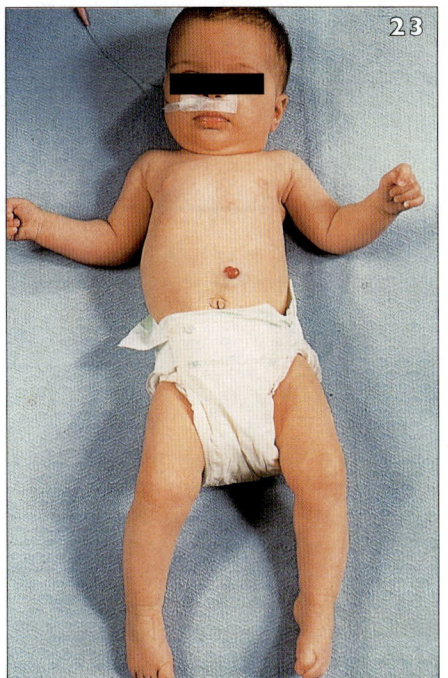

22 This patient was assaulted and complains of paresthesia over the right cheek as well as double vision (22).
i. What is a likely diagnosis?
ii. What associated injuries might there be?

23 This baby has developed slowly increasing stridor over the last month (23).
i. What is the abnormality?
ii. What would be your management of this baby?

24 A 5-year-old boy presented having passed red urine. He had complained of a sore throat the previous week.
i. What tests should be performed on this urine sample?
ii. What other investigations are necessary?
iii. What should be this patient's management?

22 i. The most likely diagnosis is a maxillary fracture. These are rare in childhood as the child's face has soft elastic bone covered by a thick layer of fat and muscle. It is not weakened by the development of sinuses and is actually strengthened by the presence of unerupted teeth in the mandible and maxilla. In late adolescence, with the adoption of a more active lifestyle, the incidence of facial fractures increases.

The paresthesia in this case is caused by compression of the infraorbital nerve. The double vision results from the prolapse of the infraorbital musculature into the maxillary sinus.

ii. Associated injuries include subcutaneous air which may result from the release of air from the maxillary antrum and malocclusion caused by a fracture/displacement of dentition.

23 i. This baby has a large hemangioma of the abdominal wall and this, together with the development of progressive stridor strongly suggests that she has a subglottic hemangioma.

ii. The hemangiomas eventually involute spontaneously but in the meantime, airway support by tracheostomy may be required. Treatment with laser and with steroids have been advocated and may hasten resolution. Such a child should be referred to the ENT surgeon without delay.

24 i. Urine should be tested (dipstick) for protein, leukocytes, nitrites, and blood. Urine should be sent for microscopy looking for the type of red blood cell morphology. Red blood cells which are glomerular in origin have a distorted shape and may be more easily recognized with phase contrast microscopy. Microscopy should also look for hyaline/granular or red blood cell casts as evidence of renal disease. Bacteria seen on microscopy are an indication of infection. Culture of the urine should be performed to rule out infection.

ii. Other tests should include: blood sodium, potassium, chloride, bicarbonate, urea, and creatinine. This may reveal hyponatremia from fluid retention, hyperkalemia from secondary renal failure, and high urea and creatinine caused by renal failure. If protein is prominent on dipstick test of urine, then serum albumin and protein tests are important. ASO titre and anti-DNAse-B and throat culture should be taken to determine etiology. This is most likely to be poststreptococcal glomerular nephritis.

The more common causes of hematuria include a urinary tract infection, glomerulonephritis, and trauma.

iii. If the investigations suggest infection, antibiotics should be started. If either hematuria or oliguria are present, the patient should be admitted for observation and antihypertensive treatment if necessary. In mild cases, the child may be discharged with follow up in 48–72 hours to check urine output and blood pressure. Eighty per cent of poststreptococcal glomerular nephritis resolve spontaneously.

25 A young girl injured her right hand while playing basketball. She complains of pain in the second digit. On inspection, she has swelling of the second digit and tenderness to palpation of the area. This X-ray was taken (**25**).

i. What is the diagnosis?

ii. What determines the treatment options?

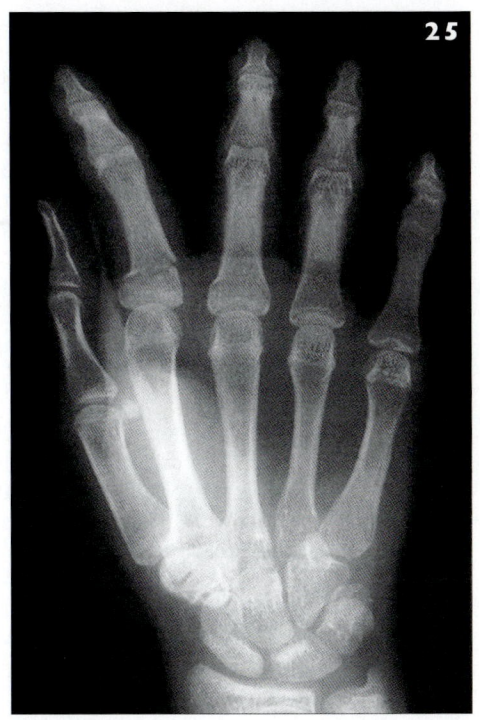

26 This 10-week-old baby has been slow and difficult to feed since birth and her mother brought her to the emergency department because she was at the end of her tether (**26**).

i. What abnormality do you notice? What is the likely diagnosis?

ii. How will the condition evolve?

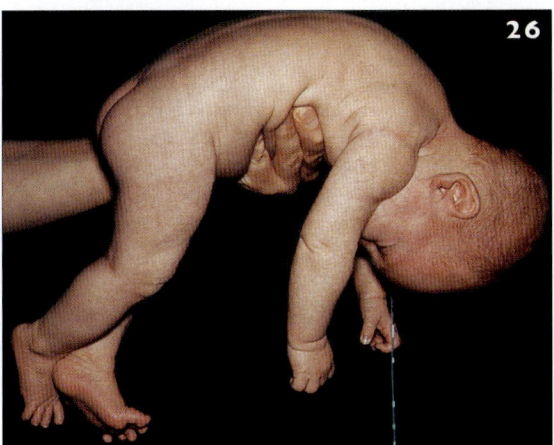

25 i. This is a shaft fracture of the proximal phalanx of the forefinger. They are usually oblique, with rotation and angulation deformities being common. The angulation deformity is easy to detect both clinically and on X-ray.

ii. The presence or absence of rotational displacement determines the treatment options. This can be assessed by noting the lack of parallel alignment of the nail beds in extension, in semiflexion or digit overlap in flexion. The injured hand should be compared to the unaffected hand as the 'normal' appearance may vary between individuals. The injury presented may be treated with closed reduction and immobilization for 2–4 weeks. However, if malrotation or displacement persists despite attempts at closed reduction, open reduction is indicated.

For phalangeal fractures affecting the ends of the proximal and middle phalanges, great care must be taken to assess the joints. Unreduced displacement of the joint surface will result in stiffness.

26 i. This baby has very poor head control for her age and has the 'floppy baby syndrome'. The poor head control was found when a developmental assessment was undertaken as part of the physical examination. A quick developmental assessment should always be part of the examination as the child is a constantly developing and both the condition with which it presents and the management of the patient may change accordingly.

The 'floppy baby syndrome' describes a baby who has marked hypotonia. There are many causes of this but it breaks down into two main groups of causes. Hypotonia associated with muscular weakness suggests a neuromuscular disorder or a spinal cord lesion whereas hypotonia without muscular weakness suggests a nonparalytic cause. The latter includes brain disorders such as cerebral palsy or Prader–Willi syndrome, chromosomal disorders such as Down's syndrome, systemic disorders such as hypothyroidism, connective tissue disorders such as osteogenesis imperfecta, and benign hypotonia.

It is important to obtain a clear prenatal, natal, and postnatal history. The birth history in this patient revealed that she had a prolapsed cord at birth and was bradycardic and slow to breathe. It is likely, therefore that she had an anoxic episode. This can set off a cascade of different pathological mechanisms leading to a wide range of possible clinical symptoms leading to any type of cerebral palsy.

ii. In the neonatal period this baby was irritable, unresponsive, and slow to feed. By about 4 months, extensor hypertonus became obvious. The baby's condition evolved until by the second year, her arms adopted athetoid movements and posture. Her legs gradually assumed the tone and posture of spastic diplegia with brisk reflexes and adductor spasticity. Bulbar palsy and poor head growth leading to microcephaly can also accompany this condition. Thus head circumference measurement is an important part of the evaluation of such a baby.

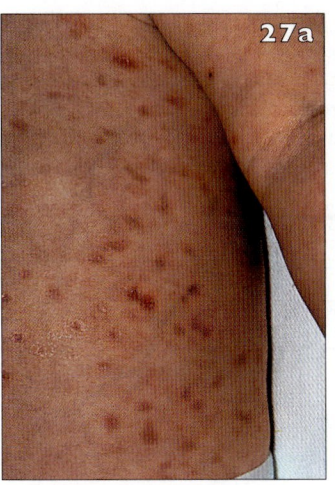 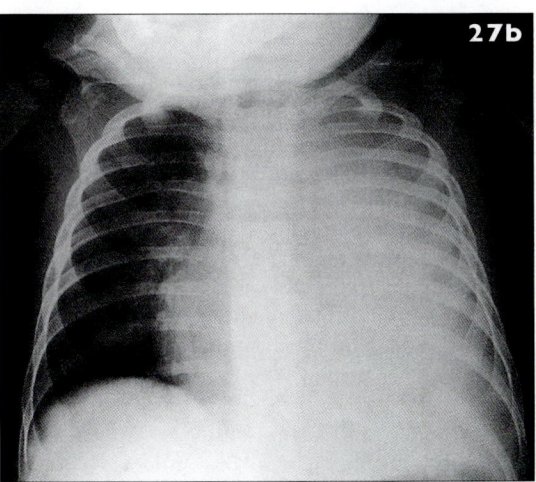

27 A 9-month-old girl presented with a 5 day history of an itchy rash, with increasing fever, tachypnea and grunting.
i. Describe the rash shown (**27a**), and suggest the most likely cause.
ii. What abnormality is shown on the X-ray (**27b**)?
iii. What two investigations would you do to confirm the pulmonary diagnosis?

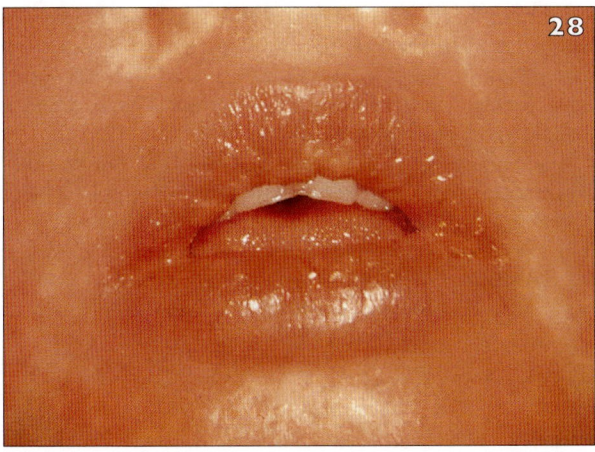

28 This 5-year-old seizure patient presents with acute onset of a rash (**28**). What is the diagnosis?

27 i. The rash is maculopapular with some crusted pustular lesions. The most likely diagnosis is chickenpox (varicella). Several days after the rash, varicella can cause pneumonia, usually in immunocompromized children. This can be fatal and therefore, exposure to varicella in this group of patients should be treated as an emergency.

ii. The chest X-ray shows opacification of the left hemithorax, with slight mediastinal shift to the right. This implies a mass or a collection of fluid in the left hemithorax. A likely cause is an empyema, due to metastatic spread of a staphylococcus or streptococcus from the skin lesions.

iii. Ultrasound of the chest will confirm the presence of fluid, and aspiration should be undertaken (preferably under ultrasound guidance) to confirm that it is an empyema. The initial management is underwater seal drainage with a large intercostal tube, and adequate intravenous antibiotic treatment. Most empyemas in childhood resolve without further surgical procedures.

28 Erythema multiforme major or Stevens–Johnson syndrome. This is a hypersensitivity reaction which, like mild erythema multiforme, may be initiated by a variety of causes including infections, including herpes simplex and mycoplasma infections, and drugs such as sulfonamides, penicillin, and anticonvulsants. If a child has a mild drug induced erythema multiforme it is important that the drug causation is noted as re-exposure can result in this severe form of the disease.

In Stevens–Johnson syndrome, the patient can present with a generalized illness with a high fever, cough, sore throat and chest pains, diarrhea and vomiting, and arthralgia. Mucous membranes of the mouth, conjunctivae, and urethra are involved. The skin lesions are initially erythematous and blotchy, beginning on the backs of the hands, feet, and trunk. Vesicles then develop within the erythematous lesions. The vesicles coalesce forming large bullae. These thin walled bullae rupture easily leading to anything from discrete cell necrosis to almost total necrosis of the epidermis. The loss of the epidermal layer in the skin results in fluid and electrolyte disturbances. The ruptured bullae are susceptible to secondary infection. The keratitis in the eye may result in infection and subsequent synechiae.

This disorder is self limiting, and untreated lasts from 6–8 weeks. However, it is potentially life threatening with a reported mortality of 5–25%. The child must be admitted to hospital for antibiotics treatment and general supportive measures. This child also needs a change of anticonvulsants. A recurrent condition can occur with reactivation of herpes simplex virus.

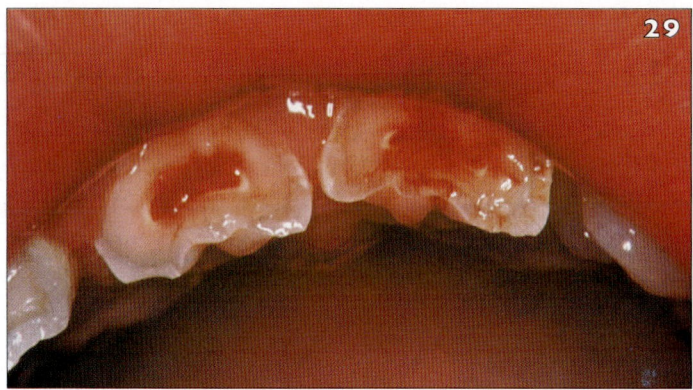

29 This 8-year-old has fractured the crowns of his upper central incisor teeth exposing the dental pulps (**29**).
i. What immediate treatment is required?
ii. What advice should be given regarding prognosis and future management?

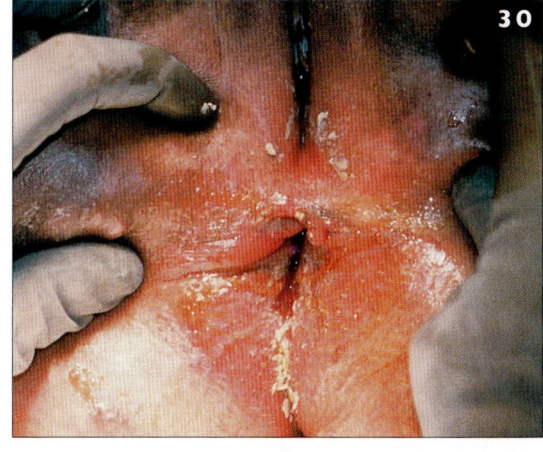

30 An 8-year-old presents at the emergency department with abdominal pain and dyschezia. She had not allowed the primary care provider to complete a genital or anal examination because of pain. The child had denied a history of abuse, but because of her complaint and unwillingness to cooperate with examination, abuse was suspected and a report to child welfare had been made. Examination under general anesthesia revealed a large perianal abscess and severely inflamed tissue (**30**). Biopsies of the inflamed tissue were diagnostic.
i. What is the cause of her illness?
ii. What extra intestinal features of this disease could present to the emergency department?

29 i. Intraoral X-rays should be taken to establish the extent of the injuries and to check that the coronal fracture is the only one these incisors have sustained. Root fractures of the teeth may require their removal. If only the crowns have fractured the exposed dental pulps must be completely extirpated under local analgesia and a sedative dressing placed over the fractured surface.

ii. The patient needs to see a dentist who can root fill the teeth and restore the fractured crowns. If the initial treatment is successful the prognosis should be excellent.

30 i. This child has perianal Crohn's disease, an inflammatory bowel disease of unknown etiology. There are many genital and anal diseases that can mimic child abuse, and although it is correct to consider the possibility of abuse when children present with genital or anal complaints, a careful medical evaluation is always in order. There are few physical examination findings that are diagnostic of child sexual abuse. The diagnosis is most often made by the history obtained from the child. Without a history of assault from the child, it would have been more appropriate to complete the medical evaluation before filing a report for investigation. Other possible causes include an association with infections, especially atypical mycobacteria, or abnormalities of the intestinal immune system.

ii. Gastrointestinal symptoms are usually present at diagnosis in Crohn's disease. However, there are also extra intestinal manifestations in 25–30% of cases and these may constitute the presenting complaint. They can cover virtually every system of the body, although the skin, joints, bone, liver, and eye are the most commonly affected.

The child can have general symptoms such as fever, weight loss, and lethargy. Erythema nodosum is the most common skin manifestation and often occurs at the time of active bowel disease and in association with arthritis.

The ocular problems include uveitis, scleritis, and episcleritis from the disease itself and raised intraocular pressure and cataracts from the treatment with high dose corticosteroids. They often occur as part of the triad with inflammatory bowel disease and joint disease.

Joint problems can include a peripheral form of hip, knee, and ankle involvement and an axial form of disease with sacroiliitis or ankylosing spondylitis.

Bone, as opposed to joint, problems include low bone density, often present at diagnosis from poor diet with low calorie and vitamin D intake, malabsorption, and bed rest. They can also result from treatment with high dose corticosteroids.

Chronic liver disease with chronic active hepatitis and sclerosing cholangitis occurs in about 1% of patients and can lead to cirrhosis of the liver and hepatic failure. Abnormal serum transaminases occur more frequently, however, at times of active disease, with medication such as sulfasalazine and 6-mercaptopurine and parenteral hyperalimentation.

In view of the protean nature of the condition, a full history and examination must be carried out. Screening investigations may show an anemia, a high ESR, hypoalbuminemia, and thrombocytosis. Further bowel investigations should include radiographic studies and tissue biopsy.

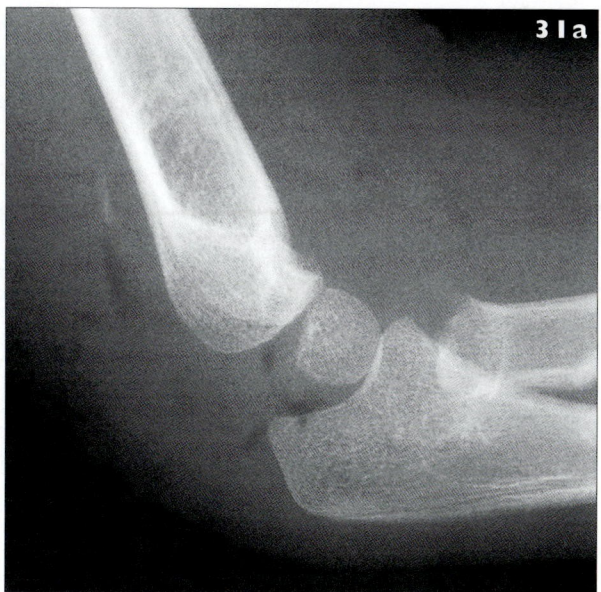

31 A 4-year-old fell off a bed and hurt her elbow earlier in the day. What abnormality is shown on the X-ray (**31a**)? What is its relevance?

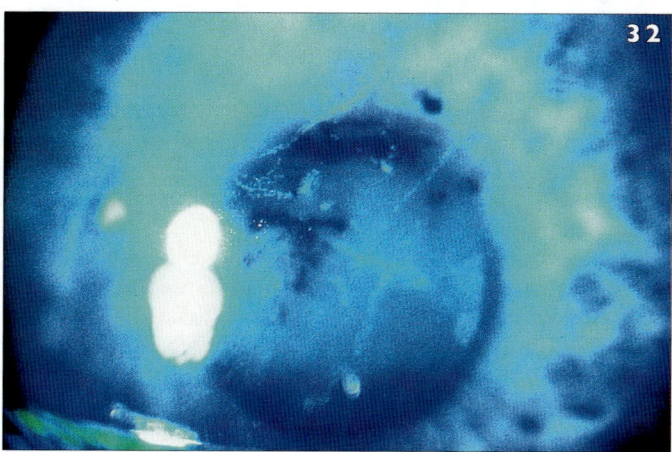

32 A linear corneal abrasion stained with fluorescein dye is shown (**32**). Where is the most likely location of the foreign body?

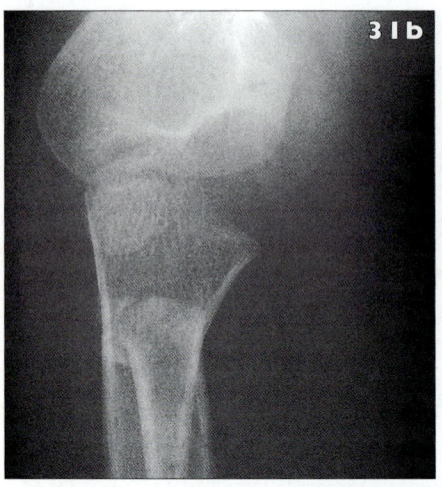
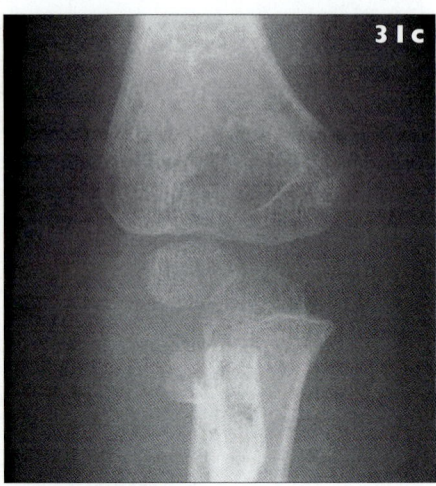

31 There is a radial neck fracture with a positive 'fat-pad sign'.

In the normal elbow fat pads lie submerged in the coronoid and olecranon fossae. When raised out of the fossae by fluid in the joint they show as dark 'billowing sails' on the lateral X-ray because the fat is more radiolucent than the surrounding soft tissues. The anterior fat pad is sometimes seen in the normal elbow (the coronoid fossa is quite shallow). Elevation of the posterior fat pad is always abnormal. In a painful elbow with a history of trauma the positive fat pad sign usually indicates an underlying hemarthrosis which in turn indicates an underlying fracture. In this case no fracture was seen on either the lateral or oblique X-rays which were originally performed (**31a, b**). As in this case, there is often an occult radial neck fracture which is readily apparent when a true anteroposterior X-ray is taken (**31c**).

32 The subtarsal area. The foreign body has migrated under the upper eyelid because of the blinking action of the eyelids. The foreign body can cause multiple linear abrasions on the corneal surface.

By everting the eyelids, the fornices and the subtarsal areas are explored as part of the routine examination.

Most foreign bodies can be removed by irrigation or gentle wiping with a wet cotton applicator, under topical anesthesia if necessary. A superficially embedded corneal foreign body is removed under topical or general anesthesia but in view of the lack of compliance with children, this should be undertaken by an ophthalmologist. Attempted removal of a deeply embedded foreign body should be avoided. The eye must be examined carefully under magnification (ideally a slit lamp biomicroscope) to determine possible perforation and removed under general anesthesia. After removal of the foreign body, topical antibiotic ointment is used until the cornea re-epithelializes.

33 A 9-month-old infant pre-sented with a fever of 6 days duration and a transient mor-billiform rash, now faded. She had shown increasing irritability and a dislike of being handled. A course of erythromycin com-menced 4 days previously by her primary care provider re-sulted in no response.

i. What abnormal sign is shown (**33a**)?

ii. Name five important dif-ferential diagnoses.

iii. Describe the clinical course of the condition.

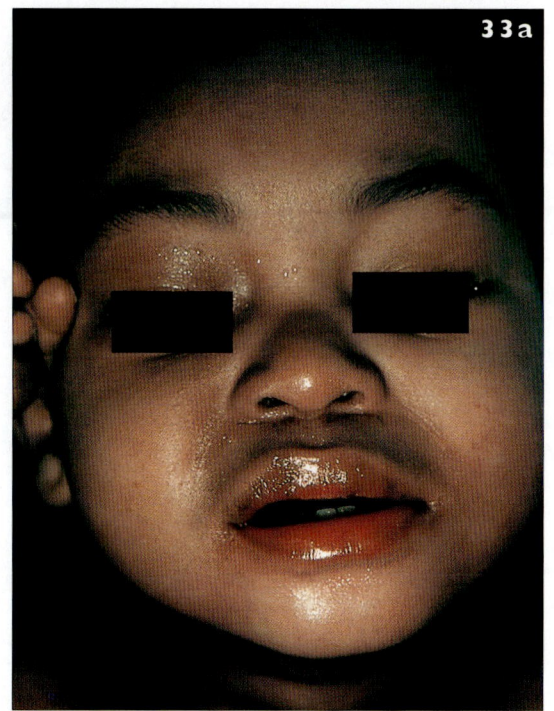

34 A 10-year-old was playing outside when he heard a noise like a gunshot. He noticed that his pants were moist and dis-covered that he was bleeding. His penile injury is shown (**34**). What diagnostic test should be performed?

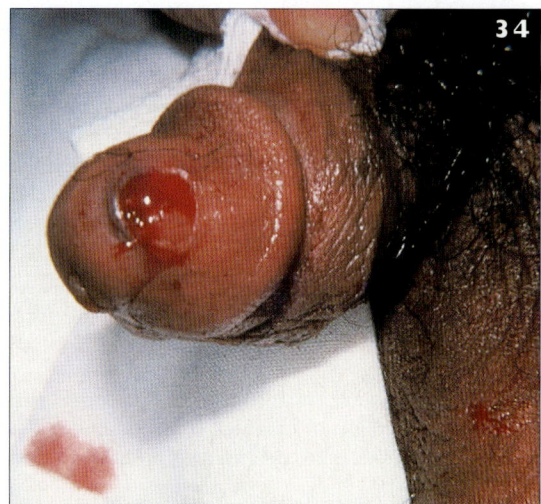

33 i. The infant has reddened swollen lips and a generally toxic appearance.

ii. Differential diagnosis includes Kawasaki disease, hemolytic streptococcal infection (scarlet fever), staphylococcal toxic shock syndrome, Still's disease (juvenile rheumatoid arthritis), glandular fever, and measles.

iii. This child has Kawasaki disease, which is of unproved etiology but is probably triggered by an infective agent and may represent an ongoing immunological response. The first week is characterized by swinging fever – which may persist for up to 30 days – injected conjunctivae, and nonulcerative reddening of the oropharynx, tongue, and lips. The palms and soles may become reddened and there may be associated nonpitting edema. There may also be asymmetrical cervical lymphadenopathy in up to 50% of cases (**33b**). In the second week of the illness, arthralgia is common and the fingers (and toes) may appear stiff and swollen (**33c**), making it difficult for the child to handle objects. In the second and third week the fingers and

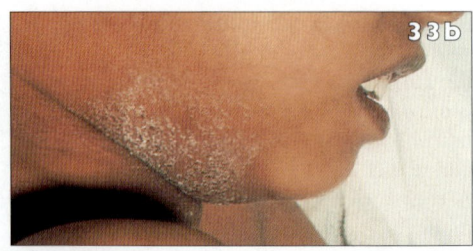
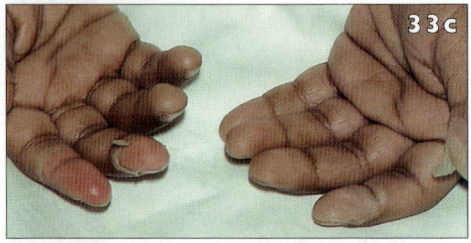
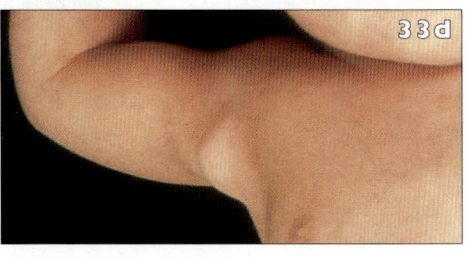

toes may desquamate, which spreads to involve the palms and soles. The fingernails may subsequently be shed. Characteristically, a marked neutrophilia develops after the first few days, followed by a steeply rising platelet count. The ESR is usually raised. Very high platelet counts are positively associated with cardiovascular problems. Cardiovascular complications, including pericarditis, myocarditis, and coronary artery aneurysms, occur in up to 20% of untreated cases. Aneurysms of peripheral arteries may also occur, as in the baby in **33d**, who developed pulsatile axillary swellings after 28 days of oscillating fever. These complications are avoided in a majority of patients if a 4 day course of intravenous gammaglobulin is given, starting within the first 10 days of the illness. The fever usually responds within 48 hours to high dose aspirin treatment. Low dosage aspirin treatment follows until the platelet count has returned to normal and the absence of cardiac involvement is confirmed by echocardiography at 6–8 weeks.

34 The findings are of an open wound to his penis. There was a corresponding exit wound and abrasion of his thigh from the bullet. The initial evaluation of the child must include a urethrogram to determine if the urethra has been fully or partially disrupted.

35 A 6-month-old Afro-Caribbean girl presented to the emergency department with a 2 week history of progressive swelling of her face, a tender jaw, and pain over her left clavicle.
i. What observations can you make on the X-ray (35)?
ii. Can you make a differential diagnosis?

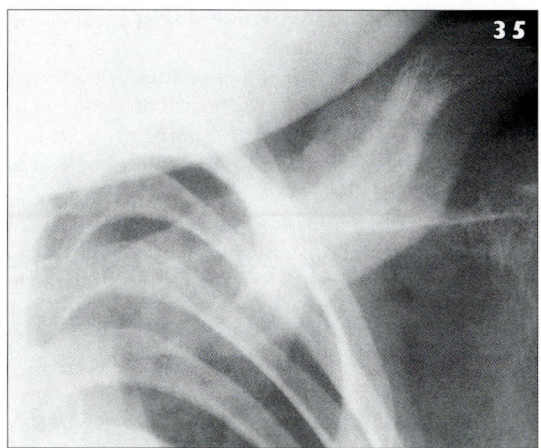

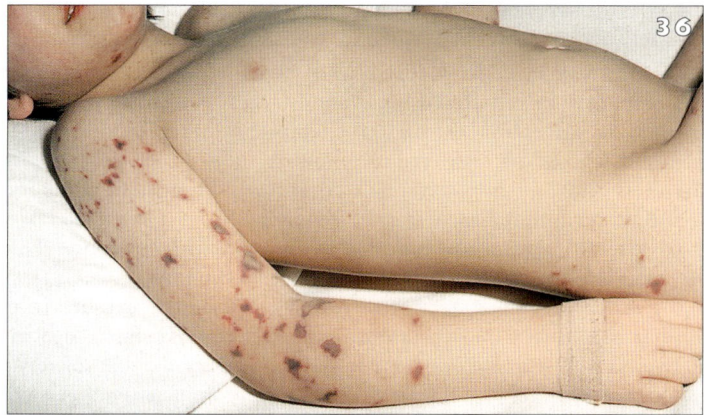

36 This child, who is the eldest of three sisters, was brought to the emergency department by an ambulance called by her parents (36). She had a head cold on the previous day but had insisted on attending her best friend's birthday party. Four hours before arriving at the hospital she felt hot, complained of headache, vomited twice, and started to be drowsy. The ambulance crew said that she was not rousable and had had a fit in the ambulance.
i. What is the likely diagnosis?
ii. The admitting doctor was engaged with another sick child and requested that the emergency doctor do a lumbar puncture before the child was transferred to the ward. Describe the investigation and management you would carry out in the emergency department.

35 i. A well-organized reaction is seen around both sides of the jaw and also cloaking the left clavicle.

ii. The appearances are those of infantile cortical hyperostosis or Caffey's disease. This is a benign, self-limiting inflammatory condition of unknown cause which presents before the age of 6 months with irritability, fever, and a nonsuppurating tender, painful swelling. Although any bone can be involved, 50% of cases affect the mandible and clavicle.

The differential diagnosis includes chronic osteomyelitis and tumor, in particular sarcomata. Chronic osteomyelitis is unlikely to present in this way or to have such symmetrical radiographic changes. Involvement of both jaw and clavicle is unlikely in tumor and the periosteal reaction is well defined, unlike that seen with sarcomata.

36 i. This child with purpura, pyrexia, and fitting most likely has meningococcal septicemia complicated by meningitis. Bacterial meningitis is essentially a disease of childhood, 75% of all cases occurring in children under 15 years of age. Children rarely have the classical signs of photophobia and neck rigidity. *Haemophilus influenzae* type B meningitis can also give a purpuric rash, but this is becoming less common as children are now being immunized against it in the United Kingdom and the United States.

ii. The initial steps of management would be according to ABC resuscitation guidelines. The airway must be secured, and breathing and circulation supported. Intraosseus access may be required if intravenous access is difficult in a shocked child. The child would be susceptible to cerebral edema and therefore, once the circulation is adequate, fluids should be restricted to minimize the risk. In addition any fits need to be controlled and any hypoglycemia corrected. Treatment with intravenous cefotaxime should be initiated early in the attendance.

Investigations would include blood glucose, culture, urea and electrolytes, bicarbonate, calcium, coagulation screen, and full blood count.

This child has features consistent with raised intracranial pressure from cerebral edema. Lumbar puncture would be contraindicated at this acute stage as the child may cone. Even a CT scan before lumbar puncture does not completely exclude a mild degree of cerebral edema. This may delay microbiological diagnosis but it is best to defer the lumbar puncture until the child is more stable neurologically, usually within 24 hours. The lack of information about the causal organism does not delay or alter antibiotic treatment as cefotaxime has a broad spectrum of action.

37 Lime burns on the ocular surface are shown (**37**). These produce a hazy cornea.

'Acid burns are usually more serious than alkaline burns.' Discuss the validity of this statement.

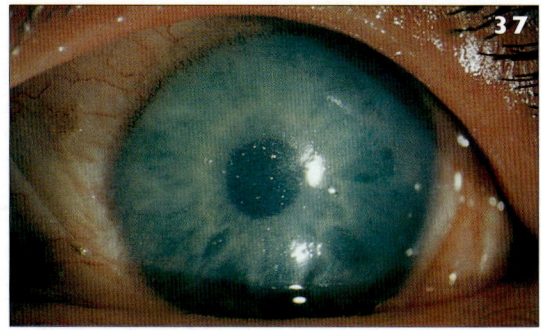

38 This child jumped off the bed while holding a pool cue in his mouth (**38**). What management would you propose in the acute stage?

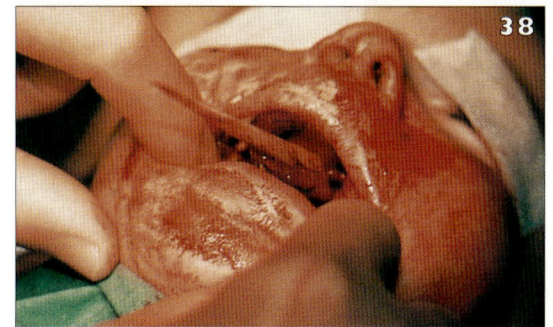

39 A 9-year-old girl presented with headache and sudden onset of left-sided weakness, lasting approximately 2 hours. When presenting to the emergency department there is no residual left-sided weakness. Her CT scan is shown (**39**).

i. What is the differential diagnosis?

ii. What abnormality is seen on the CT scan and what other investigations would you perform?

iii. What action would you take in the emergency department?

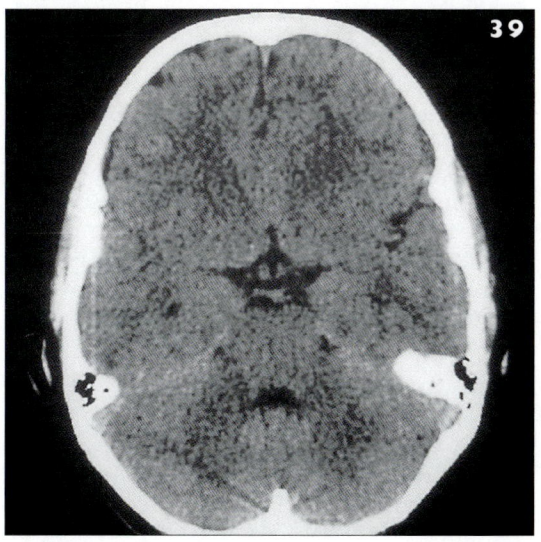

37 False. Alkalis readily penetrate the eye because they are lipid soluble. They have a prolonged effect by being held in the tissues. Their lipid solubility results in damage to other anterior segment structures such as the iris, lens, and ciliary body.

Acid injuries (except hydrofluoric acid) are more likely to be confined to the ocular surface area of contact resulting from the coagulation of tissues. This creates a barrier to further tissue penetration.

The most important immediate therapy for any chemical injury is copious irrigation with normal saline. The end point of irrigation is when the pH of the tear film is back to neutral on testing the tear film with litmus paper or urine dipstix. Any particulate matter present must be removed under topical anesthesia or general anesthesia if the child is unable to comply with topical removal.

38 The most important thing in this case is to protect the airway from obstruction by bleeding. Suction may be required and the child should be placed in the recovery position if there is any suggestion of airway impairment. Anesthetic advice should be sought without delay, as should the advice of an ENT surgeon.

The risks of this sort of injury include perforation of the palate and fracture of the skull base. In this case the pool cue was removed uneventfully under general anesthetic.

39 i. The differential diagnosis consists of:

- Hemiplegic migraine (as symptoms are associated with headache and have now almost completely resolved).
- Todd's paresis following a seizure which was unwitnessed.
- Cerebral arteriovenous malformation or aneurysm with a small bleed. This is unlikely as symptoms have resolved quickly and the CT scan is normal.
- Acute hemiplegia of childhood, a diagnosis by exclusion.

Other rare causes are encephalitis, hemoglobinopathies (e.g. sickle cell disease), and vasculitis (e.g. systemic lupus erythematosus). Most of these do not resolve so quickly.
ii. The CT scan shows no abnormality. If a seizure may have occurred then an EEG may be helpful, but usually no other tests are necessary.
iii. Treatment of this episode would consist of reassurance and explanation, as the symptoms have resolved. Discussion with parents regarding prophylactic treatment may be left to their treating physician. Propanolol or pizotifen may have benefits in preventing attacks if these are frequent or severe. Usually explanation and reassurance is all that is necessary.

40 i. What abnormalities are seen on this X-ray (**40a**)?
ii. What is the next appropriate action? What are the late complications of this condition?

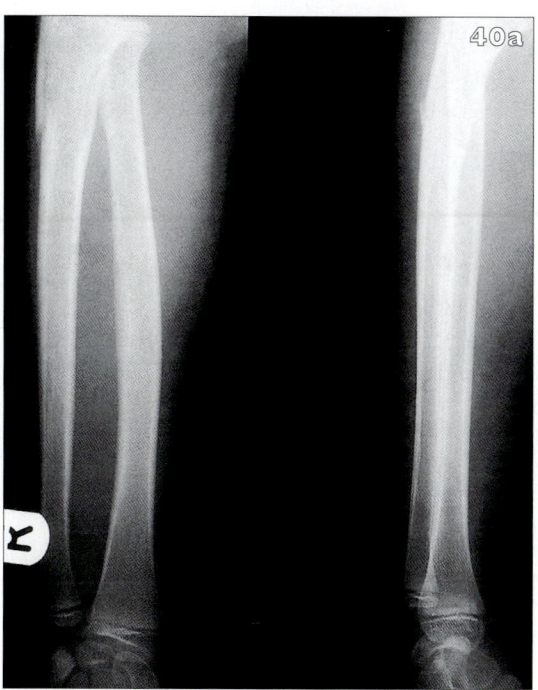

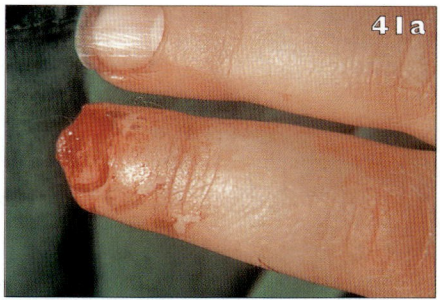
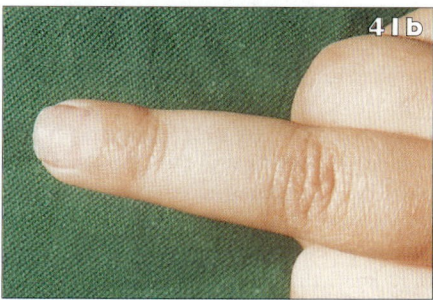

41 A child trapped his finger in the hinge end of a door. The fresh injury is shown in **41a** and the same finger 12 weeks later after treatment is shown in **41b**. Describe what you see in the fresh injury. What would be your management of this case?

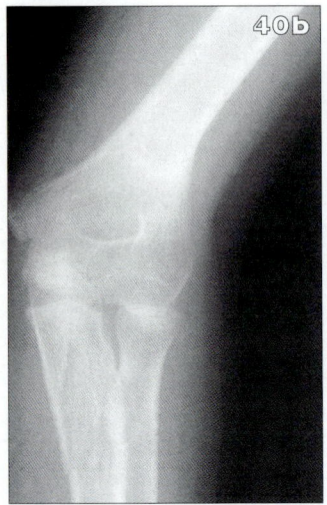 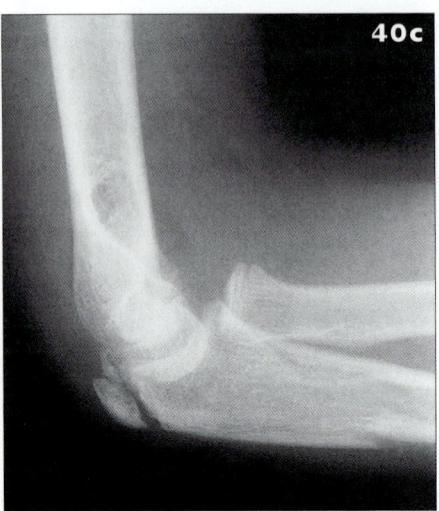

40 i. This is an angulated proximal ulnar shaft fracture with a radial head dislocation (Monteggia fracture-dislocation).

ii. It is of fundamental importance not only to obtain X-rays showing the joints at each end of a fractured long bone but to make certain that they are true antero-posterior and lateral projections (**40b, c**). In this case the ulnar fracture was identified but failure to obtain a true lateral X-ray of the elbow resulted in the radial head dislocation being missed with resultant elbow stiffness.

Beware the apparent isolated forearm bone fracture.

41 This child has lost the tip of his finger. The bone of the terminal phalanx is just visible, but the tissue loss is distal to the nail fold.

In this type of fingertip injury, with little or no bone exposure, conservative treatment gives the greatest chance of a good cosmetic and functional recovery. After thorough cleaning and debridement of any nonviable tissue, weekly dressings with an antiseptic impregnated paraffin gauze leads to healing of the finger with regeneration and remodelling of the tip. The parents and child need a careful explanation and if possible sequential photographs of a similar case to demonstrate how good the outcome will be. After the initial shock of the injury, parents often demand treatment from a plastic surgeon. This is rarely necessary.

Prophylactic antibiotics are necessary if a crush injury of the finger tip leaves bone exposed, or if the injury is associated with a fracture of the terminal phalanx as osteomyelitis is a complication of this condition.

If a significant amount of bone is exposed, then referral to a hand surgeon is necessary.

42 A 3-month-old boy presented to the emergency department with a history of being ill for 3 days and feeding poorly with occasional vomiting of milk. His parents thought he had a temperature. On examining the abdomen the lower pole of each kidney could be felt, as well as the bladder. There were no symptoms specific to the renal tract such as dysuria (crying on passing urine) or a poor stream of urine.

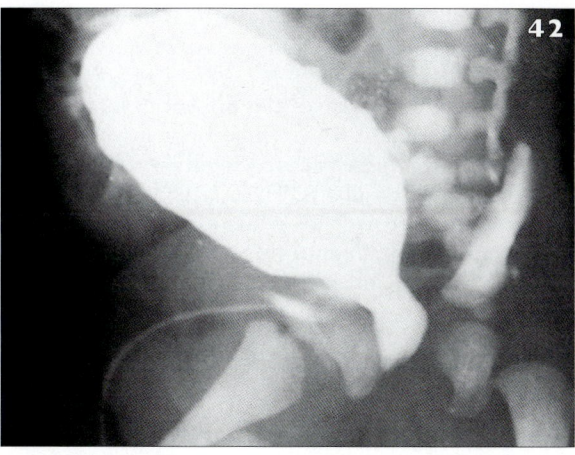

Urine culture confirmed an infection and later an ultrasound confirmed bilateral hydronephrosis and hydroureters. A micturating cystogram from the boy is shown (**42**).
i. What is the diagnosis?
ii. Are the lack of dysuria and poor urinary stream surprising?

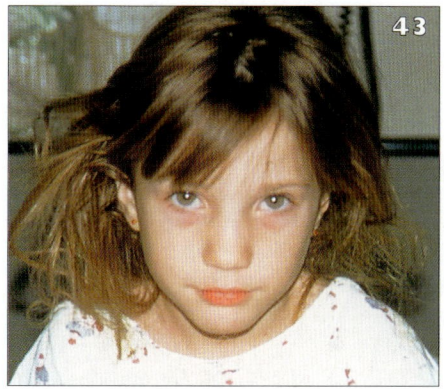

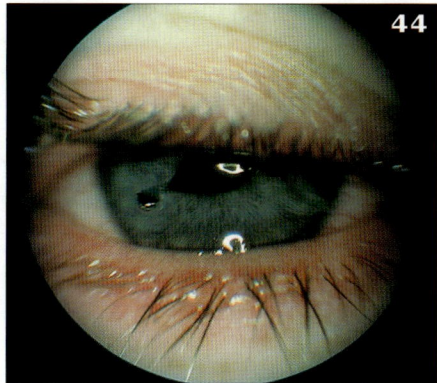

43 This child suffered a 2.5 m (8 ft) fall 3 hours ago (**43**).
i. About which injury should you be worried?
ii. What other findings could suggest this injury?

44 What does this slide show (**44**)? What type of eye drops should not be used in this condition and why?

42 i. The diagnosis is of posterior urethral valves. The typical dilated posterior urethra is demonstrated almost as far as the membranous urethra, where it finishes in a smooth curve.

ii. Posterior urethral valves can present in infancy with a urinary tract infection. The usual presentation of urinary infections in young infants is of a nonspecific illness as in this patient. A urine culture should therefore be part of the investigation of a young baby with such an illness. Dysuria is rarely noted in urinary infections in this age group and is more likely to be associated with perineal lesions. A poor stream of urine may be noted with urethral valves, but is a poor indicator of the condition.

With improved antenatal ultrasound scans the diagnosis is most commonly made as part of the follow-up of antenatally diagnosed hydronephrosis.

This child should be admitted for full investigation and expeditious management of the obstructive uropathy.

43 i. You should be concerned that this child suffered a basilar skull fracture. This child demonstrates 'raccoon eyes', which is caused by a tracking of blood from a fracture site to the loose periorbital tissue.

ii. Other findings in patients with basilar skull fractures include blood at the mastoid process (Battle's sign), hemotympanum, and CSF rhinorrhea.

Cervical spine injury can be associated with this type of fall and must be considered during the management of this patient.

In most centers, all children with a basilar skull fracture would be admitted. Recent evidence suggests that selected patients with basilar skull fracture can be discharged with appropriate home observation. However, associated neurologic findings and CSF leak are definitely indications for admission.

44 The slide shows corneal perforation with iris prolapse.

Iris tissue incarcerated in a corneal perforation with an irregular pupil should not be given dilating drops. Mydriatics dilate the pupil and may retract the prolapsed iris tissue and exacerbate aqueous humour leakage with further damage to intraocular contents. The eyelids should be gently opened without exerting pressure on the eye as this encourages further prolapse of intraocular contents through the perforating site. If a child is uncooperative then it is safer to protect the eye with a plastic shield temporarily and proceed with a formal examination under general anesthesia. Early referral to an ophthalmologist is essential.

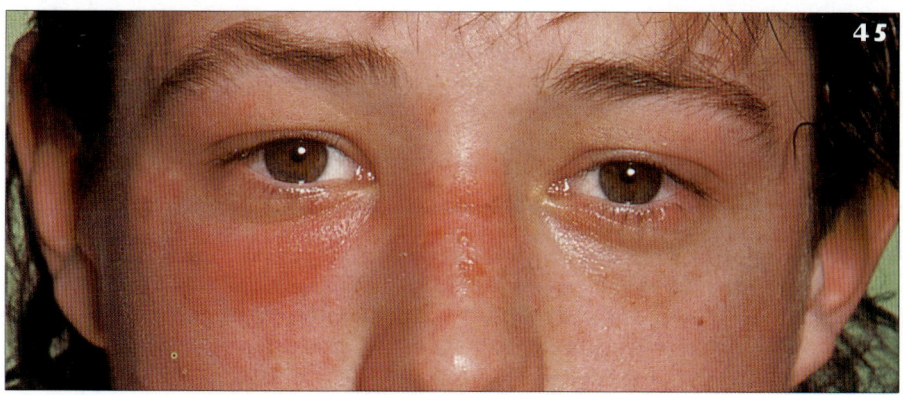

45 This boy has developed a rash below his right eye 2 days after sunbathing (**45**). It is the third time he has had this rash in the same place. What is the condition? What is the likely prognosis?

46 An adolescent, while playing soccer, caught his little finger on the jersey of a player from the opposing team. This X-ray was taken (**46**).
i. What is his diagnosis?
ii. How would you treat this injury?

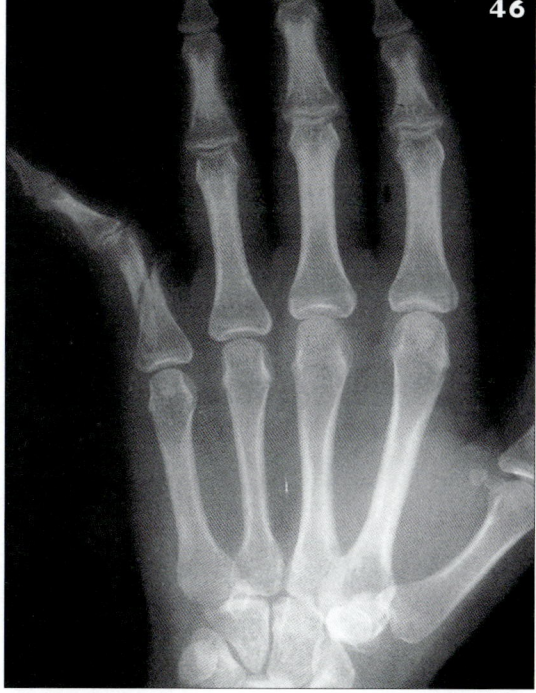

45 The patient has a recurrent herpes simplex eruption.

Herpes simplex is a DNA virus. There are two strains, *Herpesvirus hominis* type 1 and type 2. Type 2 primarily affects the genital tracts of adults.

The primary infection with *Herpesvirus hominis* type 1 in children may be sub-clinical or it may cause a variety of primary clinical conditions including herpetic gingivostomatitis or cutaneous involvement from direct inoculation of injured skin. There is also a risk that the child may autoinoculate the eye giving rise to a corneal ulcer.

After the primary infection, the virus can remain in a latent form in the tissues. It can become reactivated by certain nonspecific stimuli such as overexposure to sunlight, febrile illness, upper respiratory tract infections or surgery. The recurrent herpetic lesion presents as a crop of papules which rapidly become vesicular, usually at or near the site of the primary lesion on almost any part of the skin, mucous membrane of the mouth, conjunctivae, or genitalia. They later rupture and become crusted before resolving. Although the lesion will heal within 7–10 days, it will recur again with appropriate stimuli. Recurrences tend to become less frequent with time.

The diagnosis can be made by viral culture and occasionally by immunofluorescent staining techniques for rapid diagnosis. However, diagnosis is usually made on clinical grounds.

Recurrent herpetic infections can be aborted with a course of acyclovir started early at the time of the prodromal tingling.

46 i. The 'extra octave fracture' is a laterally (ulnar) deviated fracture of the proximal phalanx of the fifth finger. In young children with open growth plates this is often a Salter Harris II physeal fracture. In this older child it is a shaft fracture with displacement.

ii. This injury may be treated with closed reduction by flexing the metacarpo-phalangeal joint and adducting the proximal phalanx. The finger should then be im-mobilized in a splint or cast including the joint above and below the injury for 2–4 weeks.

47 This boy presented to the emergency department with a 3 week history of puffiness around the eyes and increasing weight (47).
i. What is the likely diagnosis and what investigations are relevant?
ii. Discuss the complications of the disease.
iii. What is the treatment?

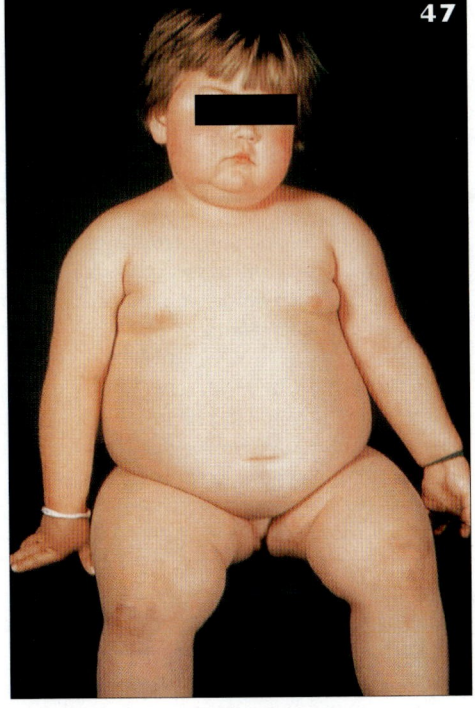

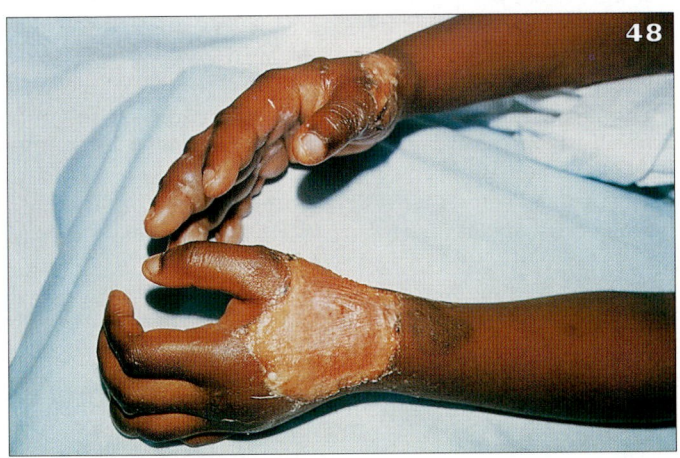

48 This child sustained these burns to his hands (48). How should he be managed?

47 i. This boy has nephrotic syndrome. This is characterized by proteinuria (>3 g/1.73 m²/day), generalized edema, hypoalbuminemia (<25 g/l), and hypercholesterolemia (>4.5 g/l). The commonest cause of nephrotic syndrome in children is minimal change disease of the kidney.

ii. Complications include: spontaneous bacterial peritonitis (pneumococcus, *Haemophilus influenzae*, and *Escherichia coli*), circulatory insufficiency (cold peripheries, poor capillary return, and postural hypotension), thromboembolism, and symptomatic edema (pleural effusions and ascites).

iii. Treatment consists of a course of high dose prednisolone, together with penicillin (as prophylaxis against pneumococcal peritonitis). Although most cases respond to prednisolone with remission of proteinuria, relapse is common, requiring further courses of corticosteroids.

48 Although injuries of the hands are rarely life threatening, they can cause considerable morbidity. The functions of the hand are so specialized that quite a small scar can cause long term problems. Assessment and management of burn injuries therefore requires considerable care and expertise.

The history of a burn must contain details of the causative agent. Scalds from baths or drinks often (although not always) cause more superficial injuries than contact burns from an iron or flame burns. It must be remembered that electrical burns can look superficial but are always deep.

The depth of a burn can be difficult to assess in a child. The parents are so upset and the child is often crying and uncooperative. However, a pink appearance and pain suggest superficial burns and a white appearance and anesthesia suggest a full thickness burn.

Any burn of a child's hand of more than a minor area requires immediate analgesia and covering with a sterile dressing and immediate referral to a burns unit.

Minor superficial burns can be simply treated with a nonadherent dressing which might consist of layers of paraffin impregnated gauze covered by layers of absorbent gauze. Although such a dressing can be quite bulky, it is well accepted by children and when applied within 6 hours of the burn has an anesthetic effect and results in a very low infection rate. Young children do not suffer from joint stiffness for more than a short period even if such dressings are used for 2–3 weeks. There are newer forms of dressings on the market for the treatment of minor burns. These need to be evaluated carefully especially in view of the success of traditional dressings.

49 i. What injury is evident in this 14-year-old boy's X-ray (**49**)?

ii. What is the most likely mechanism? Why is this injury less common in younger children?

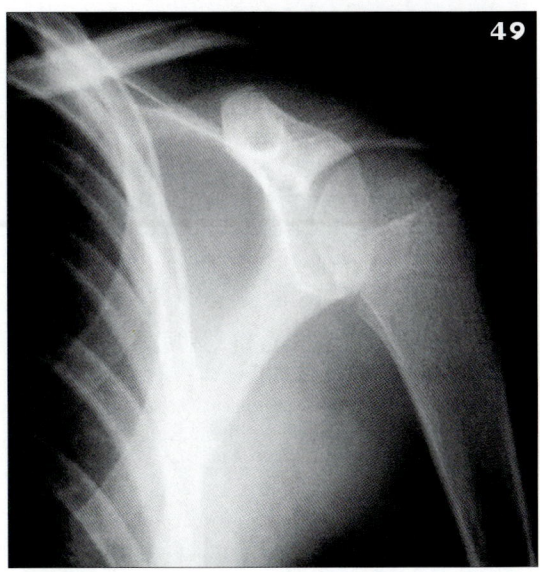

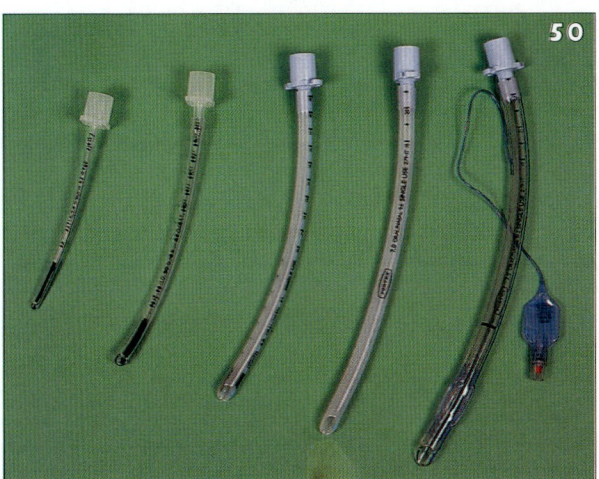

50 A 2-year-old boy was found face down in his grandparents' garden pond. He was not breathing when he was brought into the emergency department despite being ventilated by bag and mask in the ambulance. These endotracheal tubes were available for you to intubate him after clearing his airways (**50**). What equipment would you choose and why?

49 i. This child has suffered a separation of the acromioclavicular joint, as evidenced by the wide joint space between the distal clavicle and the medial aspect of the acromion.

ii. Acromioclavicular joint separation usually occurs after a direct fall onto the shoulder. It is less common in young children, who instead tend to suffer a metaphyseal clavicle fracture. Varying degrees of acromioclavicular joint separation can occur, depending on whether or not the acromioclavicular ligaments are sprained (first degree), or torn (second degree). These injuries usually respond well to immobilization with a sling and swathe. Third degree separations involve tears of the coracoclavicular ligament as well. This injury often requires surgical repair.

50 A variety of lengths and widths of cuffed and uncuffed endotracheal tubes are available. In a young child it is essential to avoid or at least minimize edema in the airways during intubation. Cuffed tubes can cause edema at the cricoid ring and shoulder tip tubes in the trachea. Red rubber tubes can also cause edema if left in too long. These should all therefore be avoided in the resuscitation of a young child and straight tubes used.

Children come in all sizes and the endotracheal tube chosen has to be the correct width and length. Simple formulae are used to estimate the size of the correct tube in a given child. It must be remembered, however, that tubes with smaller diameters than calculated should also be available if the child presents with airway obstruction from edema.

The formulae are: internal diameter in mm = (age/4) + 4.

Length for oral endotracheal tube in cm = (age/2) + 12.

Straight and curved bladed laryngoscopes are available. Straight bladed ones can be used to lift the epiglottis to prevent it obscuring the vocal folds or it can be placed short of the epiglottis and rest in the vallecula. This sort is used for babies of up to 1 year and often for children up to 5 years. In older children the curved bladed laryngoscope is used. This is designed to rest in the vallecula and therefore cause less stimulation which may lead to laryngospasm.

The cross-sectional area of the laryngoscope blade is designed to hold the tongue to the left to prevent it obscuring the airway. Inexperienced doctors may have difficulty in controlling the tongue and practice on an anesthetized patient or on a teaching model is essential.

It should be noted that it is possible to intubate a child with a laryngoscope which is too large but not with one which is too short.

In the child in question, therefore, the doctor may chose a straight or curved bladed laryngoscope and a straight endotracheal tube of internal diameter 4.5 mm (0.2 in) and length 13 cm (5 in).

51 A child presented with a pain down her arm. She had developed this rash over the previous 2 days (**51**).

i. Describe the physical signs and state the most likely diagnosis.

ii. Why should you carry out a thorough clinical examination of the whole child?

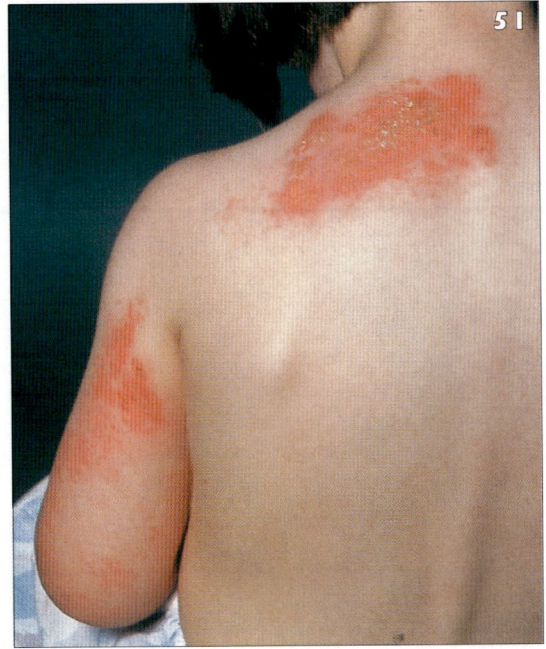

52 A child was hit in the eye by a football. Describe the condition shown (**52**), and discuss the need for pupil dilation in this patient.

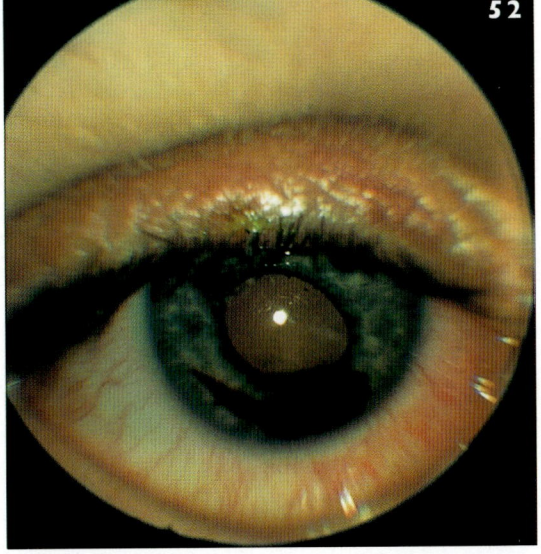

51 i. This patient has shingles, caused by the varicella-zoster virus.

In healthy children, primary infection with the virus may lead to chickenpox while secondary infection is manifested by herpes zoster (shingles). Occasionally the primary infection is subclinical. After the primary infection, the virus is latent in the sensory root ganglia of the cord and brain. It can later be activated by either local precipitating factors or by depression of immunological mechanisms by such factors as malignant disease or radiotherapy.

The herpes zoster infection can first present with mild constitutional symptoms and itching, burning or pain over a dermatome most commonly in the region of the head, neck or thorax. Some days later, the rash begins to appear as clusters of macules which develop into papules and then vesicles. The vesicles coalesce until they are bigger than chickenpox vesicles. These break and a golden crust of vesicular fluid develops. As this separates, revealing a raw ulcerated area, bacterial superinfection can occur. Resolution finally occurs, often with desquamation of the affected area.

Management usually only entails general supportive measures as in chickenpox. However, in immunosuppressed children and those with the very rare disseminated disease, parenteral acyclovir can be life saving.

Once a rash has healed, irritation and rarely neuralgia may persist for some months. Adults can be given a course of corticosteroids to reduce the risk of post herpetic neuralgia but this has not been shown to be effective in children.

ii. Conditions such as leukemia can present with shingles in a child. This girl should therefore be fully examined and have at least a full blood count.

52 The slide shows a traumatic hyphema secondary to the blunt trauma. The cause of the bleeding is the rupture of fine capillaries in the iris and/or ciliary body. The source may be sphincter tears of the iris or a tear involving the anterior face of the ciliary body, known as angle recession. It is important to dilate the pupil with mydriatics to allow a fundal view and to relieve ciliary spasm. Prompt referral to an ophthalmologist is needed.

Topical steroid eyedrops (e.g. prednisolone or betamethasone) are used to suppress an associated anterior uveitis and the patient is admitted for bed rest. At times, sedation may be needed. The use of systemic antifibrinolytic agents (e.g. tranexamic acid or aminocaproic acid) to prevent further secondary hemorrhage is controversial.

Other potentially associated anterior segment damage includes areas of iris dialysis, traumatic mydriasis caused by iris sphincter rupture, angle recession with secondary glaucoma, traumatic cataract, and lens subluxation or dislocation.

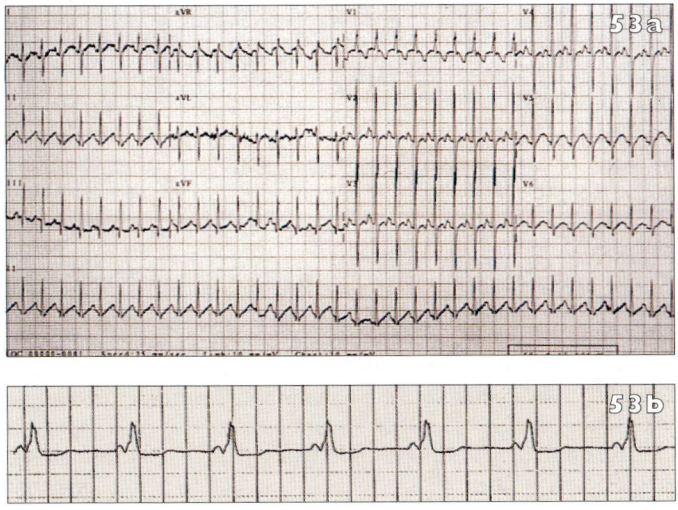

53 A 1-month-old baby presented with poor feeding, sweating, and mild tachypnea.
i. What do the ECGs show (**53a, b**)?
ii. What other investigations should be undertaken?

54 A 3-year-old child had been helping his father with some home improvements. He had a choking episode while left alone next to his father's workbench. He was well when he arrived at the emergency department and clinical examination revealed no abnormalities. An X-ray was taken.

i. What do you see in the abdominal X-ray (**54**)?
ii. What would you advise the parents?
iii. How else might you have investigated this?

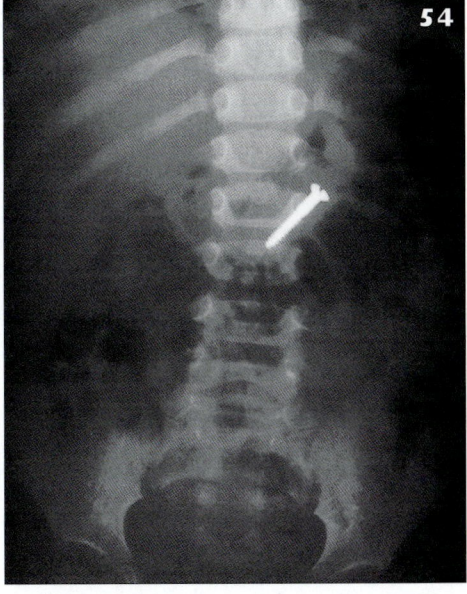

53 i. The diagnosis is supraventricular tachycardia, the commonest arrhythmia in infants and young children. The heart rate is generally over 200 beats/minute with no P waves visible on ECG and a narrow QRS complex. A circuit of conduction is set up, with premature activation of the atrium via an accessory aberrant pathway. This leads to excitation and tachycardia. The poor cardiac output if prolonged would lead to left atrial hypertension and pulmonary edema, followed by heart failure. In 80% of cases supraventricular tachycardia is idiopathic, but it may be associated with structural abnormality of the heart, e.g. atrial septal defect, Ebstein's malformation, cardiomyopathy, and mitral valve prolapse.

ii. A 12 lead ECG should be performed after reversion has occurred. This may show abnormal ventricular excitation expressed as a slur or delta wave due to early antegrade activation of the ventricle via the pathway, with a shorter P–R interval (<0.12 sec) and a prolonged QRS (>0.12 sec) as seen in Wolff–Parkinson–White syndrome. These children should not be maintained on digoxin and need to have flecainide. The blood level of flecainide should be closely monitored. An echocardiogram should be undertaken to exclude underlying structural abnormalities. Follow-up with cardiological review is necessary for all these children and long term treatment will be determined by the presence of abnormalities.

54 i. A 3.8 cm (1.5 in) screw is seen in the stomach. Most foreign bodies – even sharp objects – pass through the gastrointestinal tract completely, provided that they go past the pylorus.

ii. His parents were advised to take him home and sift his stools in the lavatory pan to ensure that the screw had passed. The screw appeared in the toilet 2 days later. If a foreign body is not passed, a repeat abdominal film is taken 3 days after ingestion, provided the child is clinically well.

Ingestion of button batteries (e.g. calculator, watch, or hearing aid batteries) needs close attention to ensure that they pass through the gut in a timely manner and that they do not open or become welded on to the esophagus or stomach, as they may cause localized ulceration from electrolytic effects.

All esophageal foreign bodies need careful monitoring and prompt referral if they become lodged.

iii. Several reports have been published on the use of a hand-held metal detector to confirm the presence and to localize ingested coins in children. The metal detector has also been used successfully on other metallic foreign bodies, but in one case an ingested needle was missed.

55 i. What is the cause of this enlarged lymph node in the axilla of a 10-year-old boy (55)? His blood count is normal. There is mild tenderness, no redness and no overlying skin rash.
ii. What other symptoms and signs might he have?
iii. How would you investigate this boy?

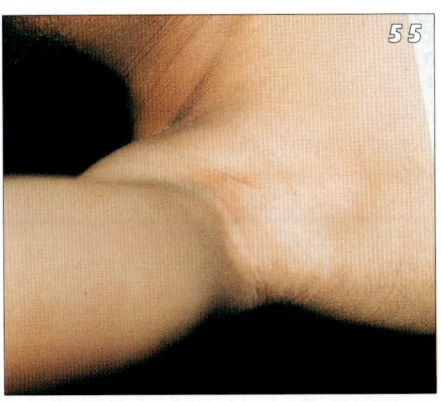

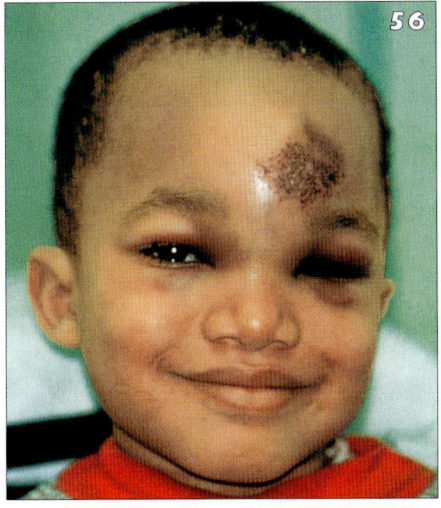

56 This child was seen on the previous day in the emergency department with a forehead hematoma after a short fall (56).
i. What is the most likely cause of the periorbital findings?
ii. What aspects of the physical examination are helpful in determining the cause? Does this child need radiographic or laboratory evaluation?

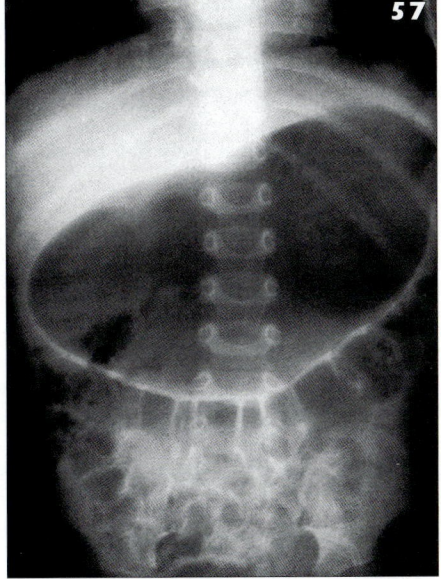

57 A 4-year-old girl was hit by a motor vehicle while riding her bicycle. She has a tense distended abdomen. A surgeon is called who recommends radiographic studies.
i. What does the X-ray show (57)?
ii. What action should be taken?

55 i. This is the chronic adenopathy of cat scratch disease. He was scratched several weeks ago by a kitten who infected him with *Bartonella henselae* organism.

ii. Children with cat scratch disease may have a more generalized form of the infection with a 'flu-like illness' including raised temperature, headaches, abdominal pain and vomiting, and myalgia. It may occasionally present as a fever with a granulomatous hepatitis. Reports have also been published of children who have blurred vision which could be unilateral. Examination revealed papilledema, a macular star, and reduced vision in one eye. The macular star looks like a firework in the eye and is formed when lipid-rich exudate leaks from the capillaries within the optic head into the subretinal space and the macular region. This neuroretinitis resolves spontaneously in 6–12 weeks.

iii. The disease occasionally gives changes in blood tests with a raised leukocyte count and ESR but these are usually normal. Routine culture of tissue from the enlarged lymph nodes usually fails to reveal *B. henselae*. An intradermal skin test of heated purulent material from the lymph node of a patient with cat scratch disease has been used in the past to aid diagnosis. However, the test is not licensed for routine use.

More recently in the USA, *B. henselae* DNA has been detected in aspirate from enlarged lymph nodes of affected children by using the polymerase chain reaction assay method. This can be performed quickly and with great sensitivity and selectivity.

Treatment with oral rifampicin and ciprofloxacin have been attempted and their effectiveness is reported to be from 73–87%.

56 i. The child most likely has a subgaleal hematoma that has begun to track into the periorbital space. It is common for hematomas to resolve by distributing to the loosely adhered subcutaneous tissue. Children with large hematomas of the forehead should be warned that they may have 'black eyes' on the next day.

ii. Physical examination should determine that there is no tenderness in the periorbital region, which can suggest an underlying orbital fracture or a periorbital infection. If there is no tenderness, no radiographic or laboratory evaluation is necessary.

57 i. The abdominal X-ray shows a markedly dilated stomach covering the entire width of the child's abdomen.

ii. Children, when traumatized, scared, anxious, or receiving artificial ventilation especially through a bag and mask, may swallow air which collects in their stomach. Not only does this make evaluation of abdominal contents very difficult, it also predisposes the child to vomiting and potential aspiration. When an oral gastric tube was placed to remove this air collection, the child's abdomen was soft, nontender, and without abnormality. The surgical consultation should be cancelled.

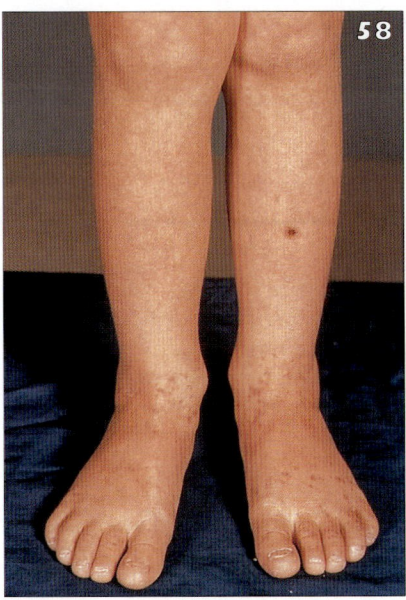

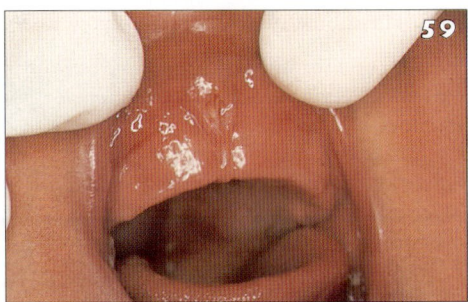

58 This child presented with tiredness and a petechial rash (**58**).
i. What is the differential diagnosis?
ii. What is the most likely cause and which investigations would confirm it?
iii. What are the common complications of this disease?

59 A 1-month-old boy was found with blood in his crib one morning by his mother. She said that she had gone out with her friends on the previous evening, leaving the baby in the care of her boyfriend, the baby's father. The father had previously taken drugs but had not had any for some time. At the time of the consultation he had a depressive illness and was on medication. They sometimes argued and he had occasionally hit her. She was sure, however, that he loved the baby and would not harm him. Physical examination revealed the finding shown (**59**).
i. What is the abnormality and how do you think this occurred?
ii. What risk factors for child abuse have you identified in the history so far?

60 A patient had pain in his neck for 4–5 days and on examination was noted to have a localized rash. Describe the skin lesion shown (**60**), and suggest a diagnosis.

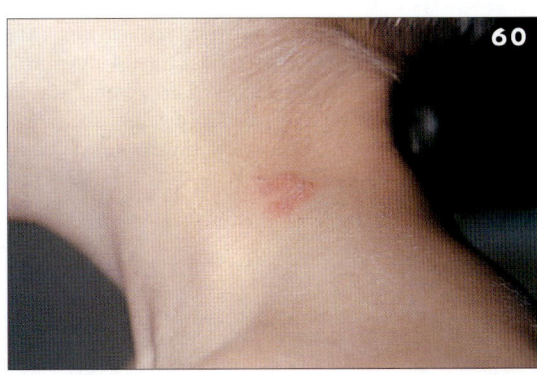

58 i. The differential diagnosis for the rash includes:

- Idiopathic thrombocytopenic purpura (the child is otherwise well).
- Henoch–Schönlein purpura (often symmetrically distributed on the buttocks and ankles).
- Child abuse.
- Septicemia (this is usually associated with fever and lethargy and the child is usually very ill).
- Acute leukemia (due to thrombocytopenia).

ii. An important cause in a child with lethargy is acute leukemia which can be confirmed with a full blood count examination. This would show a low hemoglobin and platelet count, and a high white cell count with peripheral blast cells. A bone marrow aspiration is necessary for confirmation and typing of the leukemia.

iii. Complications of acute leukemia can be life threatening and include infection, hemorrhage, and metabolic disturbances.

59 i. This is an acute tear of the upper labial frenulum. In young infants, this injury is quite specific for inflicted trauma, and may be the result of forced feeding. Frenulum injuries in older infants who are learning to walk are more commonly accidental. A careful mouth examination is an essential part of the physical examination of infants who are suspected to have been abused.

ii. This baby's family show several risk factors for child abuse. There is parental mental illness, parental substance abuse, and domestic violence, all worrying features.

This baby needs a full medical assessment and then should be taken care of in a safe place while professional workers assess the degree of risk to the child. It is likely that a lot of help and support needs to be given to the parents before the baby could be safely allowed home to their care.

60 This young man has a past history of chickenpox and has developed pain in his neck plus a skin lesion consisting of a group of vesicles. The skin lesion resembles a herpetic lesion and this boy has a very mild herpes zoster eruption. Healthy children do get herpes zoster eruptions, but they are often less severe and less extensive than 'full blown' shingles suffered by adults. The range of presentations can, therefore, range from a herpetic rash all along a dermatome to pain and a small localized eruption as in this case and even to zoster sine herpete, where the patient gets pain along the dermatome but no rash at all.

Irritation can persist for some time however mild the rash.

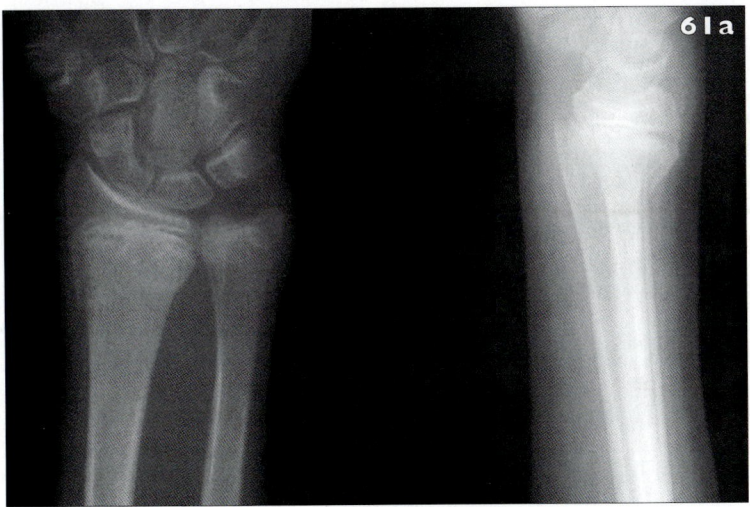

61 i. What is this injury of the distal radius called (**61a**)?
ii. Describe the classification of these injuries and their complications.

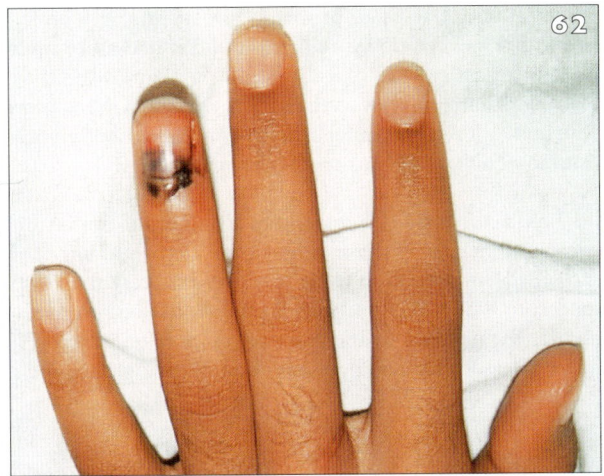

62 This 14-year-old girl accidentally closed her finger in the door at school (**62**).
i. What is your diagnosis?
ii. How would you relieve her pain?

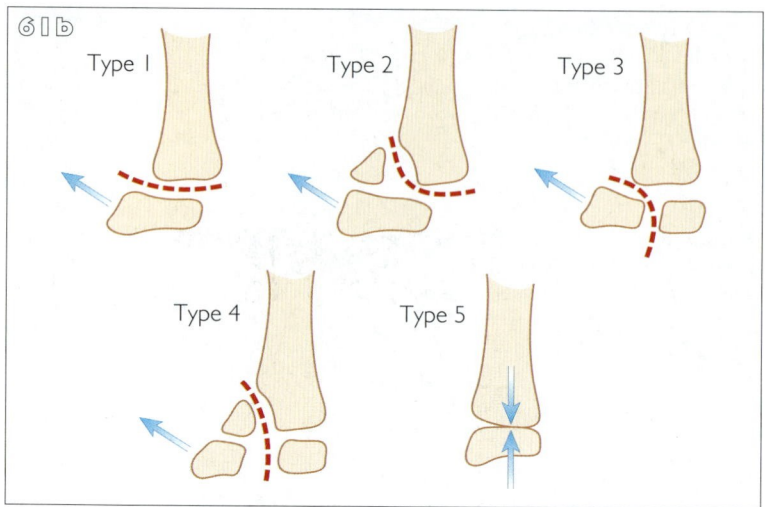

61 i. This is a fracture through the growth plate (or physis).

ii. The most widely used classification is the Salter–Harris method (**61b**).

Because the epiphysis has displaced dorsally with a small fragment of metaphyseal bone it is a Salter–Harris type 2 injury. Displaced injuries such as this require manipulation under anesthesia. This is generally easy and the reduction stable. These heal quickly in about 3 weeks and late problems are surprisingly rare.

Types 3 and 4 require careful closed reduction and if necessary open reduction and fixation as they are intra-articular.

Type 5 injuries are crushing injuries to the physis. This may lead to premature closure of the growth plate and as a result angular deformity and, or, shortening of the bone may occur. These often look quite innocuous on the original X-rays.

62 i. This child has a subungual hematoma. Subungual hematomas result from bleeding of the germinal matrix of the nail bed after a crush injury to the fingertip.

ii. Pain relief is provided by evacuation using hand held cautery (nail trephination). After evacuation, wound care with soaks and bandaging should be provided. If a hematoma completely obliterates the nail bed or the nail itself is violated or disrupted by the initial injury, there may be an associated nail bed laceration that would require repair.

63 A 3-year-old has been seen repeatedly for high fever, irritability, and conjunctivitis. He returned with a change in the skin of his hands (**63**).
i. What is the cause and what treatment should be given?
ii. What long term sequelae should be borne in mind?

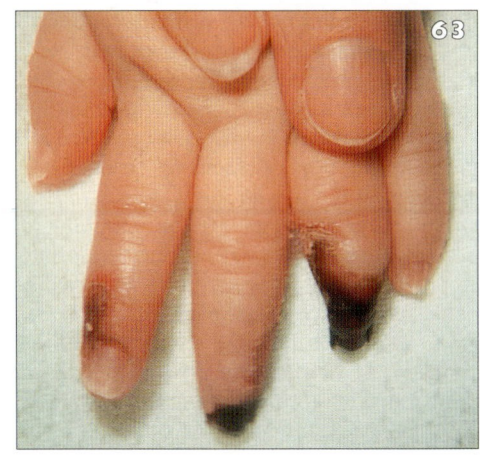

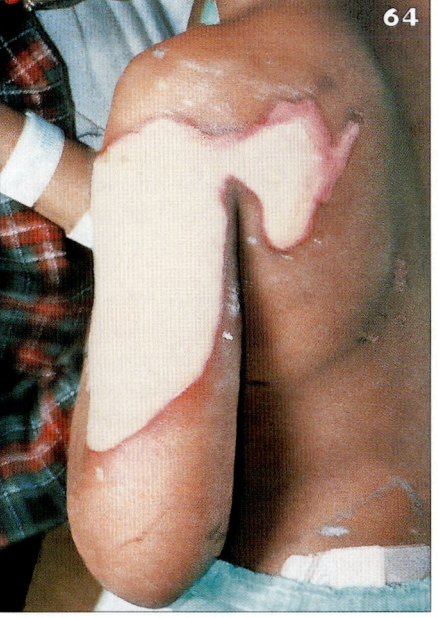

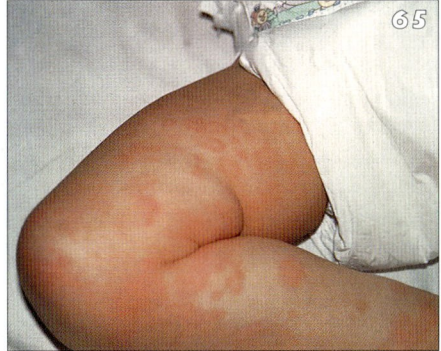

65 This 2-year-old presents with crankiness, fever and a skin rash (**65**).
i. What are the most common causes of this rash?
ii. What treatment do you recommend?

64 This 8-year-old child presented with a burn to her arm (**64**).
i. Is this a scald or a dry burn?
ii. How do you explain the distribution?

63 i. The findings of the primary condition are those of Kawasaki disease. This has a 10-fold higher incidence in Japan than in Western countries. The findings can include high fever, rash, conjunctivitis, mucous membrane involvement, and adenopathy. The children with Kawasaki disease have many different presentations as the disorder is a vasculitis that can involve many different organ systems. Most deaths occur within the first 2 months of diagnosis. Irritability is a common finding. The child's vasculitis is evident in the fingers showing endarteritis. The child must be admitted to the hospital and treated with intravenous immunoglobulins and high dose salicylates.

ii. Cardiology consultation must be obtained to rule out the early cardiovascular complications such as coronary aneurysms. However, there is increasing recognition of the possibility of ischemic heart disease in adults as a consequence of childhood Kawasaki disease. Young adults who have had Kawasaki disease have been reported from the United States and Japan with coronary artery obstruction and coronary aneurysms, without atherosclerotic changes.

64 i. A dry burn.

ii. The child's sibling lit her clothes, causing the flame burns to the child's arm and back. The child removed her clothing by pulling it down her body, thus avoiding her face.

Burns are the second most frequent cause of accidental death in children. House fires are the most common fatal cause and particularly affect the 1–4 year olds. Death is usually related to smoke inhalation and respiratory failure, hypovolemic shock, renal failure, and overwhelming infection.

Although the majority of pediatric burns are due to scald injuries, flame, contact, chemical, and electric burns are also frequently seen. Most pediatric burns are the result of preventable accidents, but may also be due to child maltreatment. Abusive burns are more common in infants and toddlers and can be caused by any of the above mechanisms.

65 i. The term erythema multiforme refers to a spectrum of diseases from erythema multiforme minor to Stevens–Johnson syndrome (erythema multiforme major) to toxic epidermal necrolysis. The majority of patients have erythema multiforme minor. There can be many underlying causes of erythema multiforme, including a wide range of organisms, such as bacterial infections, histoplasmosis, mycoplasma, herpes simplex and almost any drug. The disease is uncommon under the age of 3 years.

The rash of erythema migrans in Lyme disease can look like the herald patch of erythema multiforme. Occasionally there can be multiple lesions in Lyme disease.

ii. Erythema multiforme is an acute self-limiting disease characterized by this rash with 'target' or 'iris' lesions in conjunction with mild systemic symptoms, including fever, arthralgia, and minimal to no mucosal lesion. Therapy is aimed at providing comfort with analgesics, antipyretics, and antipruritics. In addition, any underlying cause of the rash should be identified, such as antibiotics for a streptococcal infection.

66 A 5-month-old male presents with wheezing and respiratory distress.
i. After stabilization a chest X-ray is undertaken. What is the most probable diagnosis based on this X-ray (**66**)?
ii. What should the initial management be?

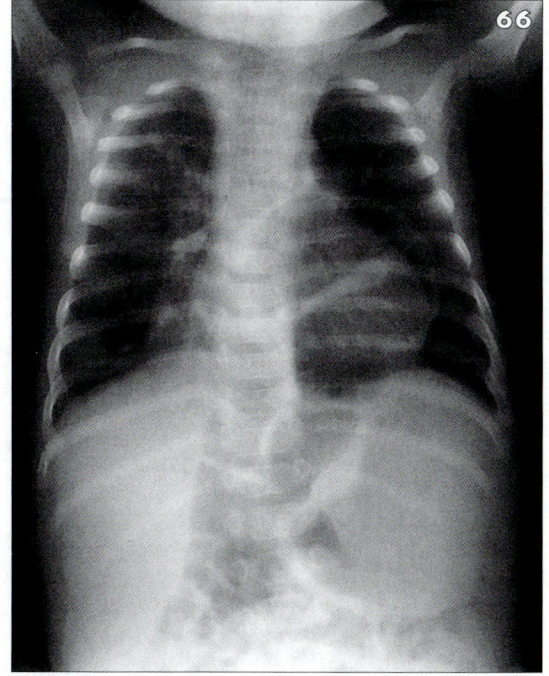

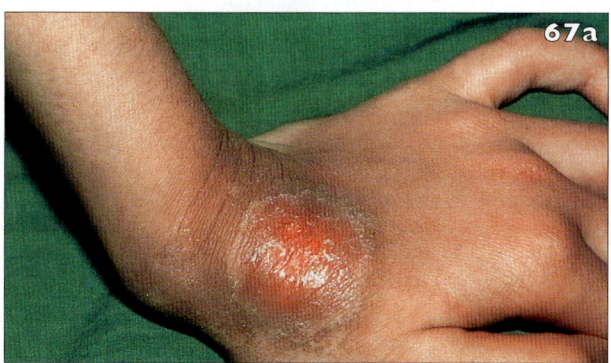

67 This 9-year-old Asian child who had immigrated 3 months earlier, presented with a lesion on the wrist (**67a**). This had been present for 3–4 weeks and had been previously diagnosed as due to trauma.
i. What are the differential diagnoses?
ii. What is the likely pathogenesis?

66 i. The most likely diagnosis is a diaphragmatic hernia. This defect of the hemidiaphragm usually occurs on the left. It can be associated with heart defects and gut malrotation but is more usually associated with severe pulmonary hypoplasia. Where the hernia is the only abnormality, the presentation may be delayed until the baby is several months old.

Although diaphragmatic hernia may be diagnosed before birth by fetal ultrasound, it is usually diagnosed just after birth. As the baby swallows air, the small bowel in the chest expands and the mediastinum shifts, compressing the unaffected lung. The baby develops respiratory distress.

ii. Following stabilization of the ABC, a nasogastric tube should be placed and surgical consultation obtained.

67 i. The differential diagnoses are:

- *Mycobacterium tuberculosis.*
- Low grade pyogenic infection with *Staphylococcus aureus*, *Haemophilus influenzae*, or *Salmonella* species.
- Atypical mycobacterium.
- Syphylitic skin infection.
- Malignancy of bone.

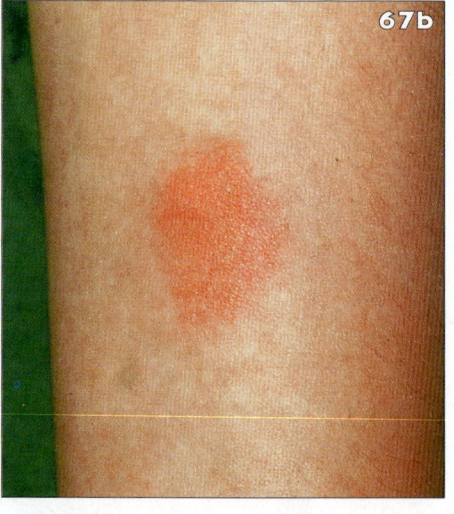

ii. A primary tuberculous infection is likely to have passed without treatment during the previous 1–3 years. The lesion may start as an endarteritis in the metaphysis of the long bone, where the blood supply is rich. Bone is progressively destroyed by cold abscess formation, which results in swelling and a cystic bone lesion (visible on radiography). This may lead to infection of an adjacent joint. A history of trauma is common, which may activate or merely draw attention to an underlying lesion.

Tuberculous skin lesions may also present as a tuberculous chancre. This is primary cutaneous tuberculosis that occurs 2–3 weeks after inoculation of *M. tuberculosis* at the site of injury on the skin or, at times, to the mucous membrane. Common sites are the chin, nose, lips, limbs, and genitalia. It is a tuberculous granuloma with caseating necrosis, starting as a reddish brown papule that gradually enlarges and ulcerates, leading to an indolent, firm, sharply demarcated ulcer. There is associated regional adenopathy and occasionally lymphangitis. *M. tuberculosis* can be isolated from the skin lesion and from the regional lymph nodes.

The child's Mantoux test was positive, indicated by skin induration of more than 5 mm (0.2 in) (**67b**).

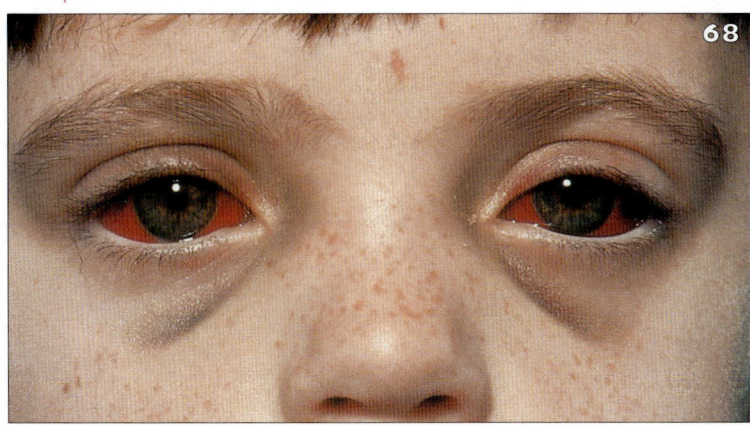

68 A girl was brought to the emergency department at midnight by her grandmother with whom she lived. The grandmother said that the girl had gone to bed alright but by midnight was found in bed looking like this (**68**).
i. What questions should the examining doctor ask in the history?
ii. What has happened and what is the likely cause?

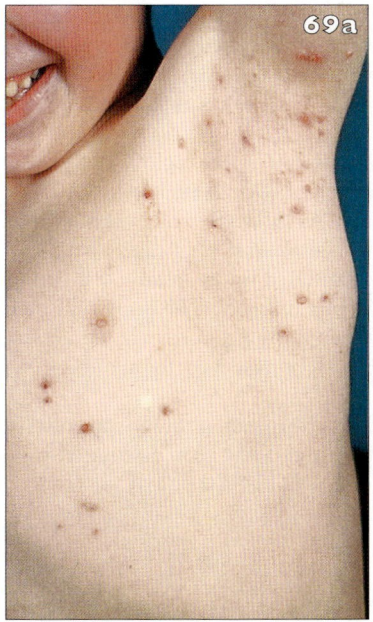

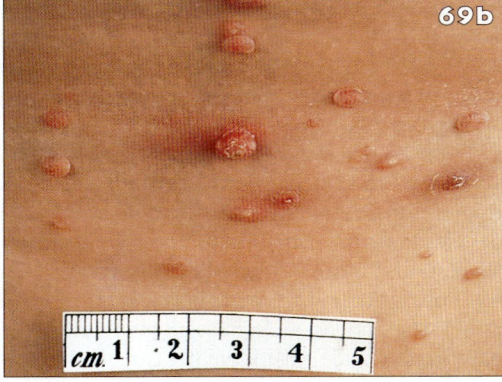

69 This 3-year-old presented to the emergency department with a rash which had been present for several months (**69a, b**). One spot had started to bleed.
i. What is it?
ii. What is the natural history and treatment of this rash?

68 i. The examining doctor should take a full pediatric history including a review of all the systems and a history of any recent accidents. A social history should also be taken.

This child had a 3 week history of a cough which was particularly bad at night, came in spasms, and ended either with a whooping inspiratory noise or with vomiting. She had whooping cough.

ii. Whooping cough can be caused by any one of three organisms, *Bordetella pertussis*, the commonest cause, *Bordetella parapertussis*, or *Bordetella bronchiseptica*. No cross immunity develops between types.

This infection can occur at any age, but its presentation can vary with age. After an incubation period of 7–14 days, the catarrhal stage is characterized by an upper respiratory tract infection-type illness with a cough lasts approximately 2 weeks. After this the paroxysmal stage occurs. In older children this takes the classical form described in this patient. However, in young babies this phase can consist of episodes of choking, or apnea without a paroxysmal cough. Whooping cough must therefore be considered in the differential diagnosis of apnea in an unimmunized baby.

Complications of whooping cough are becoming less common. They consist of epistaxes, fits, secondary lung infections, pneumothoraces and spontaneously resolving petechiae of the face, and subconjunctival hemorrhages. The latter has happened in this case.

69 i. This is molluscum contagiosum caused by a large pox virus. It occurs equally in both sexes, mainly in the second half of the first decade of life when 2–3% of children have been found to have lesions. The differential diagnosis includes warts or herpes simplex. Molluscum contagiosum has discrete papular umbilicated lesions which can be singular or multiple. They can occur mainly on the trunk, axilla, face, and diaper (nappy) area. They can be spread by scratching when they appear in a linear arrangement.

ii. These lesions last for many months. They are not particularly contagious but can be annoying and can bleed when traumatized. The onset of a delayed hypersensitivity reaction and spontaneous resolution may be heralded by scaly red rings around old papules. Lesions usually resolve spontaneously if left alone but may take up to 2–3 years to disappear. An inflammatory reaction can be initiated to the lesion by Burrows solution, cryotherapy, or picking out the central caseous material. The body will then attack the lesions and cause them to resolve. Cryotherapy or curettage is usually painful and will leave a small scar. Treatment should be reserved for troublesome lesions only.

It is more common in patients with AIDS, those with other immunosuppressive disorders, and those receiving immunosuppressive therapy. It has been associated with various nonsexual modes of transmission such as swimming and sharing of towels.

70 A 13-year-old was a pedestrian involved in a motor vehicle accident.
i. Describe the injury (**70**) and outline the strategy for the initial management in the emergency department.
ii. How might this child's pain be relieved?

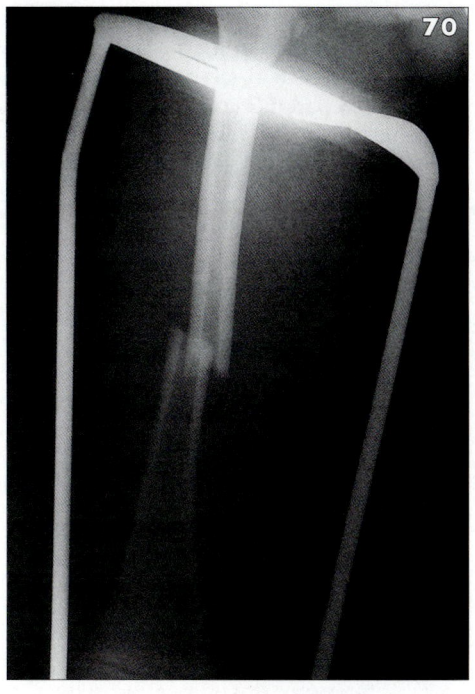

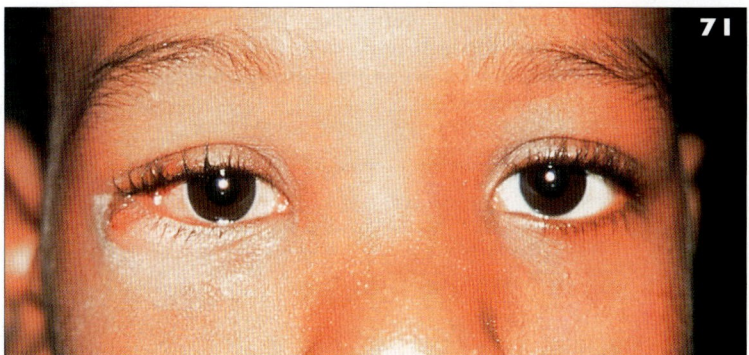

71 This 8-year-old boy presents with the complaint of swelling and redness in his right eye (**71**).
i. What is the diagnosis?
ii. What is the treatment?
iii. What closely related condition may have the same presentation as this case?

70, 71: Answers

70 i. This child has a displaced mid-diaphyseal fracture of the femur. The leg injury was clinically obvious. This is a high energy injury and attention is first directed to ABC assessment with cervical spine immobilization as detailed in APLS and ATLS training. Once stabilized the patient is more fully examined in the 'secondary survey'. The right thigh was obviously deformed and the distal pulses were examined and found to be intact. Should there be any evidence of foot ischemia in spite of adequate cardiac output it must be assumed that the femoral artery is occluded at the level of the fracture and the limb pulled straight and held in a Thomas' or other traction splint. Radiographs are not needed at this stage.

ii. A femoral nerve block just below the inguinal ligament provides significant pain relief while applying the splint but remember to check sensation before performing the nerve block. Failure to restore circulation demands urgent orthopedic and vascular referral. The nerve block and fracture splintage often provides satisfactory initial pain relief but if not a titrated intravenous dose of morphine (0.1 mg/kg) can be given. This is not contraindicated in those with head injuries.

In this case the child had a head injury and was unconscious, requiring endotracheal intubation and intensive care. The vital signs were stable and there were no other injuries. The neck was immobilized in a hard collar and the femoral fracture was treated using an external fixator.

71 i. This patient has a stye or hordeolum, which is a staphylococcal abscess occurring at the base of the eyelashes. There is localized swelling, redness, and pain.

ii. The removal of an eyelash may promote drainage of the pus. Treatment consists of warm compresses in conjunction with a topical antibiotic preparation, both four times per day. The eye drops should be continued for some days after the hordeolum subsides.

iii. A Meibomian cyst is initially a noninflamed lipogranulomatous swelling in the Meibomian glands of the eyelid which drain near the conjunctiva. This can become infected. If the condition does not resolve spontaneously, the gland may need excision.

72 What are the risks with this type of injury (**72**)? Discuss the principles of prevention and management of such an event.

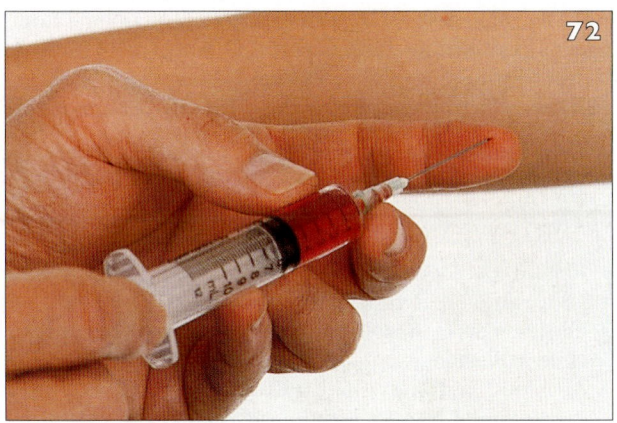

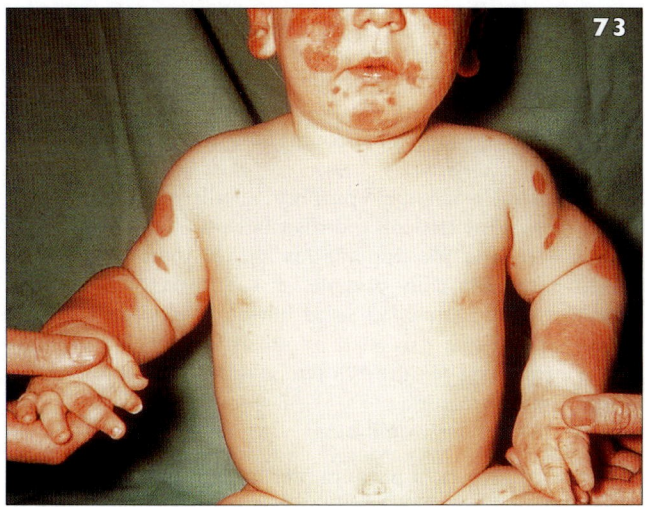

73 A 12-month-old child had a recent upper respiratory illness and fever. He awoke with this purpuric rash (**73**), but was well and had no meningeal signs. All his investigations were normal, including full blood count, ESR, blood culture, and bleeding and clotting screens. An autoimmune screen revealed normal antinuclear antibodies, rheumatoid and precipitin antibodies.

i. What is the most likely diagnosis?
ii. What is unusual about the presentation in this case?
iii. What would you consider in the differential diagnosis and how would the investigation results help to confirm your diagnosis?

72 The main risk of a needle-stick injury is infection with a blood transmissible agent. Examples include hepatitis B, hepatitis C, and HIV. Prevention is based on universal precautions with all blood products.

Avoid penetrating injury with potentially contaminated sharp objects:

- Dispose of all sharp objects in approved sharps containers.
- Needles should not be recapped or removed from syringes manually.

Avoid contact with blood or potentially infected bodily fluids:

- Regard all blood and bodily fluids as potentially infectious.
- Gloves should always be worn when handling blood or blood products.
- Gloves, masks, aprons, and goggles should be worn in clinical situations where a child is bleeding.
- All blood and body fluid spills should be cleaned up immediately and disposal of waste should be into infectious waste bags.

Management of a needle-stick injury requires base-line serum from the recipient at the time of the injury in case it becomes necessary to relate the injury to the subsequent development of a blood borne viral infection. The source and recipient should be tested for hepatitis B. If the recipient is not immunized and the source is HBsAg positive, hepatitis B immunoglobulin should be given within 48 hours of the incident and a full course of immunization should follow. The decision regarding investigation for HIV follows individual counselling and discussion.

73 i. This child has Henoch–Schönlein purpura, an allergic vasculitis.
ii. In this case the age of the patient and distribution of the rash are atypical as the case involves an infant and the upper body rather than the classic distribution. Henoch–Schönlein purpura usually presents at 4–8 years of age and usually affects the extensor surfaces of the arms, legs, and buttocks, but can involve any site. The classical purpuric rash can be preceded by an urticarial rash and painful swollen joints may be the presenting feature. Other possible symptoms include abdominal pain, testicular pain, and hematuria.
iii. Other conditions to consider would be:

- Child abuse – this is a picture of purpura, not bruising.
- Sepsis – the full blood count, ESR and blood culture would be abnormal.
- Bleeding diathesis – bleeding and clotting screens would show abnormalities.
- Idiopathic thrombocytopenic purpura – low platelet count.
- Connective tissue disease – abnormalities in the autoimmune screen.

There are no findings to support any of these alternative diagnoses.

74 This young boy had a 'school booster' injection into his left upper arm 3 hours previously (**74**).

i. What immunization was he given and which component is the most likely to have caused the reaction?

ii. What advice would you give about further immunizations?

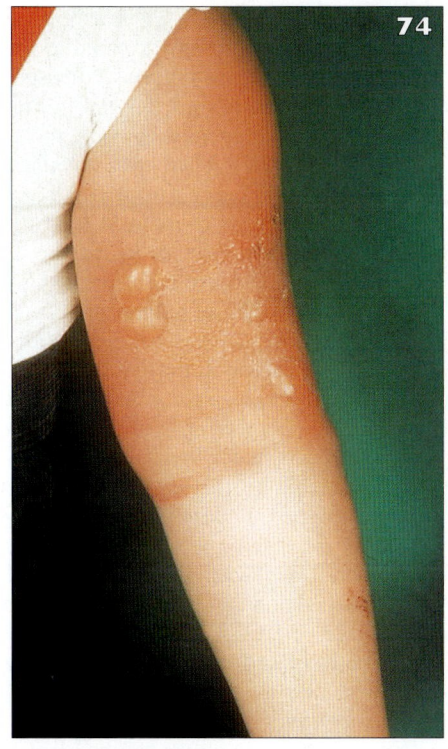

75 A girl put her hand under a fence while trying to reach for a dog. While pulling her hand out, she cut her second and third digits (**75**). She now complains of not being able to make a fist.

i. What is her injury?

ii. How would you identify it on inspection?

iii. What is the treatment for this injury?

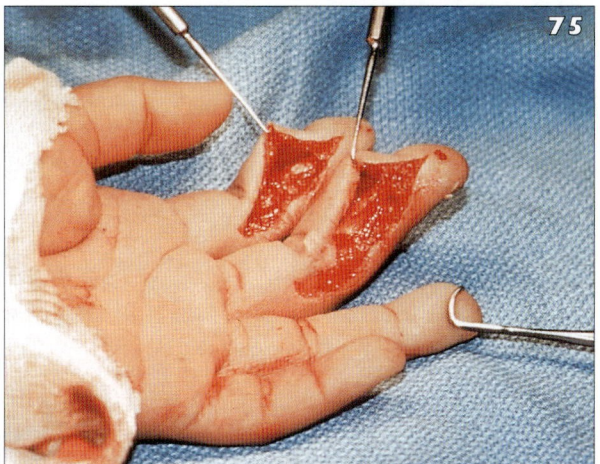

74 i. The boy has been given a booster dose of adsorbed diphtheria and tetanus vaccine. He is likely to have reacted to the tetanus portion of the vaccine.

Normal tetanus prophylaxis consists of a primary course of triple vaccine containing diphtheria toxoid, tetanus toxoid, and killed *Bordetella pertussis* by intramuscular or subcutaneous injection at 2 months of age, followed by two further doses at monthly intervals. Thereafter, a child has a further dose of tetanus and diphtheria toxoid at school entry and a further reinforcing dose of tetanus and low dose diphtheria vaccine for those aged 13–18 years.

Adverse reactions can occur to the tetanus toxoid and are more common if an individual has had more than five doses in total. The local reaction, the commonest, usually consists of pain, redness and swelling around the site of the injection and lasts for several days. A localized firm nodule may result at the site of immunizations which are given too superficially. Less commonly, general reactions of headache, lethargy, malaise, myalgia, and pyrexia may occur and, rarely, there may be anaphylaxis and peripheral neuropathy.

ii. This boy has had a local reaction only to his immunization. Local reaction is not an absolute bar to further immunization but this should only be undertaken in a setting equipped to deal with an anaphylactic reaction. The primary care provider should be informed and the boy and his mother should be instructed to inform any doctor who may wish to give the boy further immunization in the future so that appropriate action can be taken.

75 i. She has lacerations to the flexor tendons of her second and third digits. This is the commonest mechanism of flexor tendon injury. Occasionally closed rupture may occur, sometimes secondary to a fracture.

ii. The nature of the injury can be identified on examination by noting the disruption of the normal cascading appearance of the fingers at rest. The tendons must be assessed individually. Laceration of the flexor digitorum profundus alone leads to flexion at the proximal interphalangeal joint but not at the distal interphalangeal joint. Laceration of both flexor tendons leads to flexion at the metacarpal phalangeal joint but not at either interphalangeal joint. A partially lacerated tendon may give tenderness on resisted flexion and may snap completely some days after the initial injury.

iii. All flexor tendon lacerations need referral to a pediatric hand specialist and operative repair.

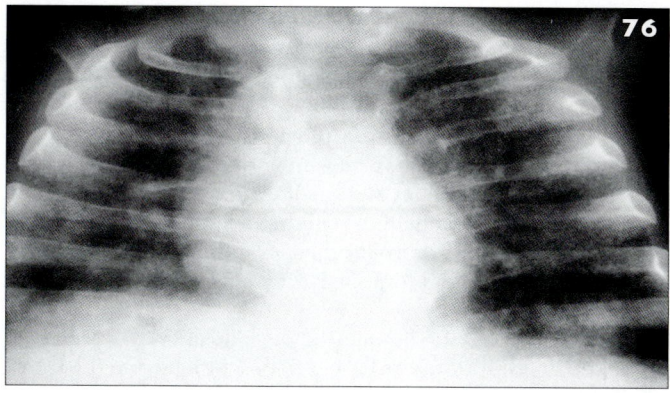

76 A 9-month-old child was brought to the emergency department as he had been ill for some time. His parents were becoming increasingly worried because he had a persistent fever despite treatment from his primary care provider. A chest X-ray was requested (76). What do you see?

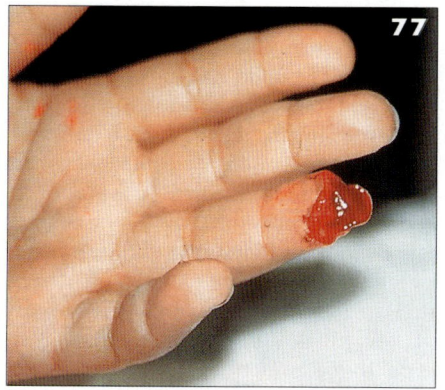

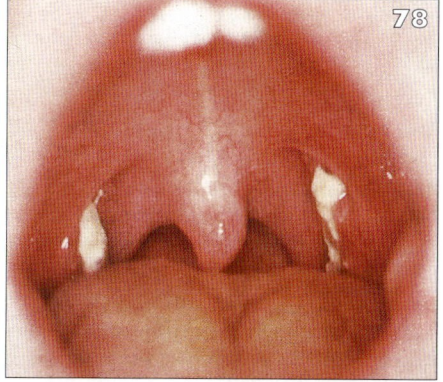

77 This 10-year-old boy had a metal gate close on his finger (77). How would you treat this?

78 This 13-year-old girl had a febrile illness, a sore throat and difficulty in swallowing (78). She has a generalized rash.
i. What is the likely diagnosis?
ii. What other clinical features might you elicit on clinical examination?
iii. How would you diagnose and manage the condition?

76 The chest X-ray (76) is a lordotic chest film, which accounts for the unusual appearances of the ribs. There is a calcified gland in the left side of the neck, and a very fine background nodular pattern throughout both lungs – like the appearances of 'millet seeds' or a snow storm in the lungs. These are features of miliary tuberculosis. In this case, calcified glands from previous tuberculous cervical adenitis are also present. The primary complex may be seen with a small parenchymal lesion with caseation of the regional lymph nodes and calcification.

It is useful to examine the optic fields of children who have chest radiographic signs of miliary tuberculosis, to detect choroid tubercles. Other lesions that may be present include osteomyelitis, arthritis, and (especially in younger children) meningitis.

77 Treatment for fingertip soft tissue injuries depends upon the degree of injury and the age of the child. Children aged 12 years or younger have better chances of adequate healing with secondary intention. This tuft amputation is without exposure of bone and therefore can heal by secondary intention after irrigation and debridement of any nonviable tissue. A nonadherent dressing should be applied with follow-up arranged within 48 hours. If, on closer examination a significant amount of bone is found to be exposed by the injury, and there is no senior doctor in the emergency department with special expertise, a pediatric hand surgeon should be involved in the care of the child. Management options of an injury with bone exposed range from conservative management to fingertip composite graft to local advancement flaps.

78 i. The child has an exudative pharyngitis with a white membrane covering the pharynx. There are also fine petechiae of the palate. The child has infectious mononucleosis, transmitted by saliva. Individuals are commonly infectious before, during, and for 6 months after infection. In Western countries it is usually a disease of school children and young adults but in central Africa almost all children are infected by the age of 3 years. Other possible underlying causes include group A streptococcal infection, diphtheria and severe infectious herpes simplex pharyngitis.
ii. Most children with infectious mononucleosis are not severely ill. In addition to the symptoms displayed by this child they might have enlargement of lymph nodes, particularly the epitrochlear ones, splenomegaly (50%), and tender hepatomegaly (30%). Perceptual distortion of space and size, known as 'Alice in Wonderland' syndrome or Bell's palsy are rarely present. This child was prescribed ampicillin for her sore throat. This will have predisposed her to the rash.
iii. Blood tests often show leukopenia, atypical lymphocytosis, a positive monospot (slide agglutinin) test, and raised liver transaminase and gamma-glutamyl transferase enzymes. Most children are managed at home with symptomatic treatment only. However, children with very severe disease or dangerous complications need admission. These can include respiratory obstruction from grossly enlarged tonsils and pharyngeal edema, neurological complications such as convulsions, meningitis, encephalitis or Guillan–Barré syndrome, or myocarditis, interstitial pneumonia, pancreatitis or orchitis. Splenic rupture, usually associated with minor trauma can also occur.

79 Injuries to the cervical spine are rare in children, but they are potentially lethal. In order to ensure that you do not miss X-ray signs of these injuries you must have a system for looking at the X-rays of the cervical spine. Describe the system you use using the X-ray shown (79).

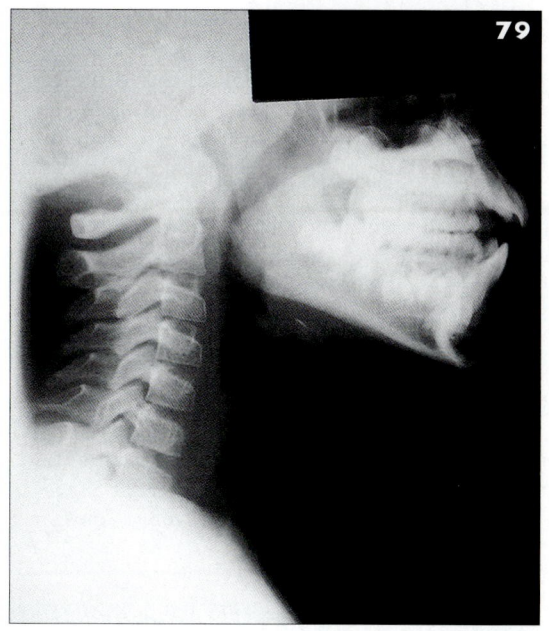

80 This previously healthy 15-year-old girl presents with rapid respiratory rate, paresthesia of hands, feet, and mouth, and posturing of her hand (80), after attending a rock concert.
i. What is the acute management?
ii. What are the differential diagnoses?
iii. What follow-up should be arranged?

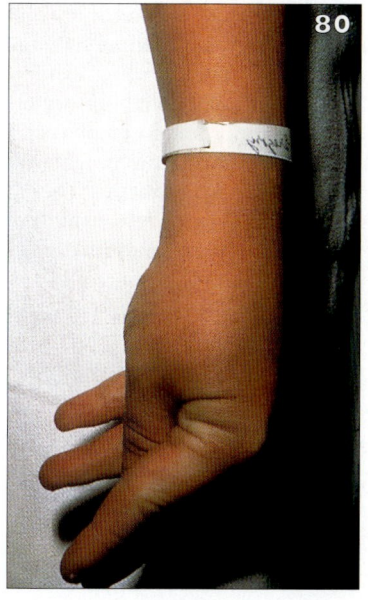

79 An example of a systematic approach to checking cervical spine X-rays follows.

First, count the vertebrae – all seven should be seen together with the top edge of the first thoracic vertebra. Unless this is the case a cervicothoracic injury cannot be excluded and the X-ray must be repeated if necessary with arm traction or as a 'swimmers' view in order to demonstrate the C7–T1 junction. Remember that when one spinal injury is seen a second spinal injury (C1–sacrum) will be apparent in up to 10% of cases.

The vertebrae should be stacked one on top of the other with a gentle lordotic curve. Trace lines down the fronts and backs of the bodies looking for a step indicating subluxation. Similar lines can be traced down the posterior elements of the spine. At the atlantoaxial level the gap between the front of the odontoid process and the back of the anterior arch of the atlas should be no more than 4.5 mm (0.2 in) in children.

A retropharyngeal soft tissue shadow is always seen anterior to the vertebral bodies and this expands with hematoma if there is an underlying injury. The normal width is difficult to quantify but it is wider over the lower cervical spine and should not be wider than the adjacent vertebral body at any level.

Finally trace around each vertebral outline looking for cortical irregularities suggesting fracture.

80 i. This patient is suffering from hyperventilation. Immediate treatment is to correct the lowered $PaCO_2$ by having the patient re-breathe into a bag.
ii. Differential diagnosis can include response to severe pain, diabetic ketoacidosis, hypocalemia, drug ingestion (e.g. salicylates), and organic CNS disorders. Patients with underlying respiratory problems (e.g. asthma) may present with hyperventilation and be mis-diagnosed as having acute asthma. These patients usually have normal peak flow meter readings and good air entry and minimal added sounds on auscultation. Extensive laboratory tests are not required in most cases.
iii. It is important to emphasize that the patient has control over the production of symptoms. This is often achieved by voluntary overbreathing and careful education by the emergency doctor. There should be psychiatric follow-up as counselling and supportive therapy are usually necessary to discover the sources of psychological disturbances experienced by the child.

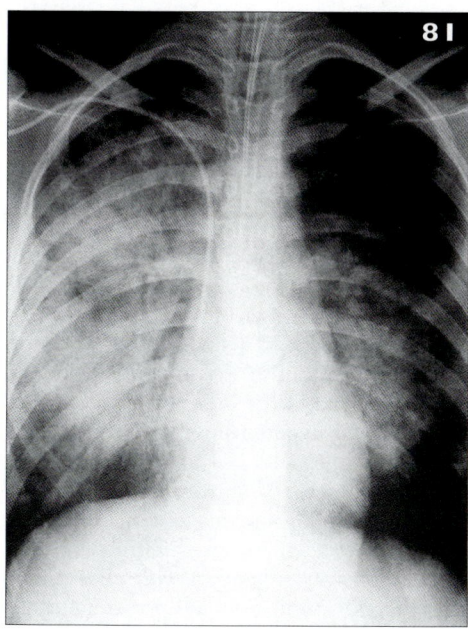

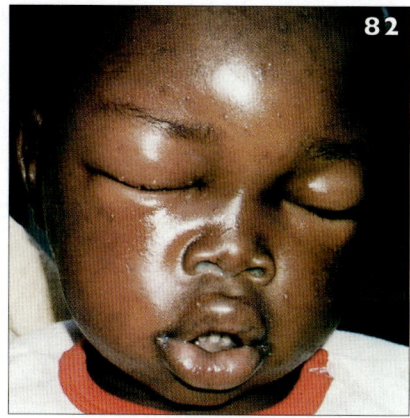

82 This baby was covered in bee stings when she presented to the local health care clinic in Africa (**82**). On examination she had too many bee stings to count. Her lips and eyelids were becoming edematous. Her pulse was 110 beats/minute and her blood pressure 90/50 mmHg (12.0/6.7 kPa). She had a respiratory rate of 40 breaths/minute and was beginning to develop a wheeze.
i. What should the immediate management be?
ii. Why might this case become more relevant in other countries?

81 A patient was referred from a local ski area because of head injury and a short period of loss of consciousness. No other injuries were reported or expected on the information given by the referring personnel.
i. What does the X-ray show (**81**)?
ii. What should be done?

83 A 6-year-old Asian boy who had immigrated 6 months previously presented with a high spiking fever, marked leukocytosis, generalized lymphadenopathy, and gross hepatosplenomegaly (**83**). What are the three main major groups of differential diagnoses?

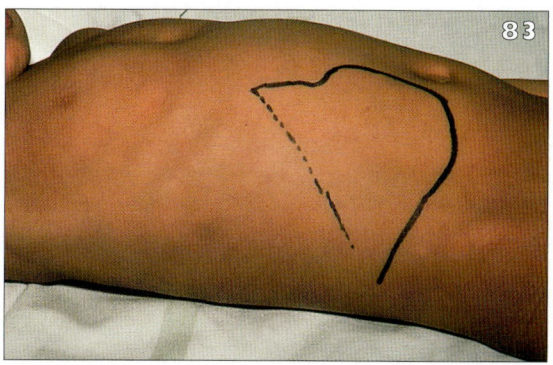

81 i. The chest X-ray demonstrates bilateral pulmonary opacities. These could result from aspiration or pulmonary contusion. Pulmonary contusion occurs relatively frequently in children in blunt trauma. They have pliable and mobile ribs and contusion to the lung parenchyma can occur without rib fracture and even without chest bruising. The blunt trauma is transmitted to the lung where it ruptures pulmonary capillaries allowing blood to fill the alveoli and preventing gaseous exchange.
ii. Pulmonary contusion or aspiration pneumonia suggests potentially significant pulmonary parenchymal disease. Supplemental oxygen and positive pressure ventilation with adequate pressure support are often necessary for recovery.

82 i. The baby was developing anaphylactic shock with onset of airway impairment due to laryngeal edema and the development of shock. This is caused by acute vasodilation and increasing capillary permeability leading to loss of fluid from the intravascular space. The anaphylactic reaction is usually dose dependent and occurs within 30 minutes of exposure to the agent. Delayed hypersensitivity up to 10 days from the injury can also occur after bee stings.

Treatment for mild urticarial reactions would consist of antihistamines with or without steroids. However, in this more severe case, full anaphylactic management became necessary. The airway was managed with oxygen via an endotracheal tube together with nebulized salbutamol. The circulation was supported with intravenous colloids and intramuscular adrenaline, which relieves vasodilation and prevents further release of cell mediators from the mast cells and the basophils. Intravenous antihistamines and hydrocortisone can also be given.
ii. African bees can be particularly aggressive. They were introduced into Brazil in 1956 and mated with the fairly docile European bees to produce a hybrid, African honey bees. These are more defensive and aggressive than European bees and respond to even slight disturbance of their nests by sending out thousands of bees. Colonies of these hybrids are gradually moving northwards through the American continent and several deaths have already been reported.

83 The three main groups are:

* Malignancy, e.g. leukemia, lymphoma, histiocytosis X, hepatoblastoma, metastatic tumors such as neuroblastoma, Wilm's tumor, and gonadal tumors.
* *Mycobacterium tuberculosis*, i.e. lymphohematogenous spread.
* Other unusual infections, such as disseminated fungal infections.

In this form of tuberculosis the Mantoux test is usually strongly positive and the response to treatment good. In this child it proved extremely difficult to make the diagnosis and he was initially thought to have disseminated malignancy of the reticuloendothelial system.

Tuberculosis should always be considered early in the differential diagnosis of an ill febrile child without a clear cause.

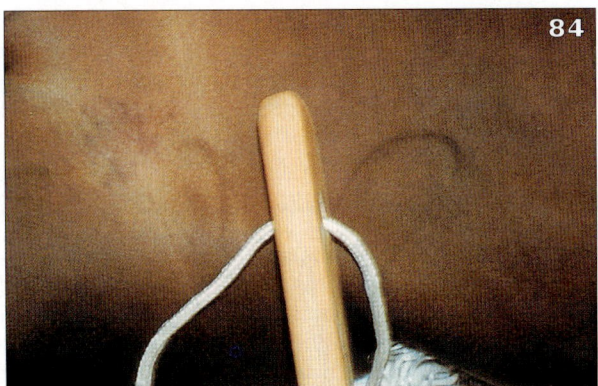

84 A 2-year-old child was said to have slipped in the bath tub. He was comatose when he arrived at the hospital. His physical examination revealed old curvilinear marks on his abdomen (84) and retinal hemorrhages. The history seemed suspect as the emergency paramedics noted that the child was not wet when they arrived at the house. Child abuse was suspected and a CT scan of the head was ordered.

i. What might you see on the initial CT scan?

ii. What injuries describe 'shaken baby' or 'shaken impact' syndrome?

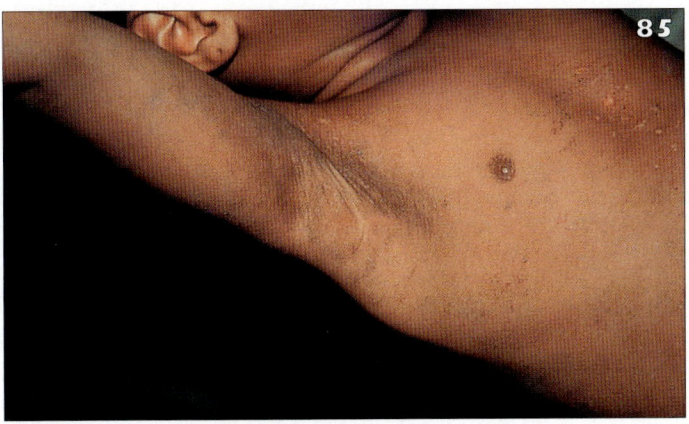

85 This 3-year-old boy presents with a rash which he has had for the past 3 weeks (85). His mother has been using calamine lotion and oatmeal baths. He seems to be getting worse and now his sister has a rash.

i. What is your diagnosis?

ii. What treatment do you recommend?

84 i. This child had signs of acute injury on the CT scan with subdural blood present in the posterior interhemispheric fissure and along the cerebral convexity. It is formed by the tearing of the bridging meningeal veins and is usually associated with severe underlying brain contusion. Only 30% of subdural hematomas in children are associated with a skull fracture. The site of any fracture is not a good guide to the position of the hematoma. In 75% of cases the bleeding is bilateral.

The signs on the CT scan can vary. Early on, cerebral edema (loss of grey–white differentiation) may be the only change.

ii. Shaken baby syndrome or sudden impact syndrome usually presents in young babies under 3 months old. However, it has been reported in older children of up to 2 years of age. The children usually present in a coma. They may have a bulging anterior fontanelle or fixed dilated pupils. Bilateral retinal hemorrhages are often present and can lie anteriorly and be difficult to find on direct ophthalmoscopy.

Debate has centered around whether these children have been shaken violently or whether there has to also be impact to cause the intracranial bleeding. The incidence of impact injuries has been reported as over 60% in one series of 48 cases. Experiments on subhuman primates suggests that shaking alone can cause the pathological findings in young babies with incomplete myelination and a greater proportion of water in the brain. In older children, impact causing great deceleration forces may be more significant than shaking alone. In nonaccidental injury, there are often other associated signs of assault. A skeletal survey is needed in all these children to detect new or healing fractures of long bones or ribs.

85 i. The chronicity, distribution and symptoms in other family members help with the diagnosis of scabies – an infestation with *Sarcopes scabiei*. The primary lesions of scabies include papules, vesicles, pustules, and burrows that represent invasion by female parasites. The typical distribution of these involves the web spaces of the hands and feet, axillae and creases of the arms, wrists, and groins.

Secondary lesions result from the intense hypersensitivity reaction to the parasites and occur approximately 1 month after infestation; lesions include allergic urticarial reaction to the parasites, eczema, excoriation, and infection. These are often the most prominent lesions present at diagnosis and are distributed on the trunk and limbs.

Young children and infants often have an atypical distribution of rash including the head, face, palms, and soles. The irritation of the chronic infestation may result in poor feeding and failure to thrive.

Diagnosis is usually made from the physical signs but where it is in doubt it can be confirmed by the isolation of a mite or an egg from burrow scrapings.

ii. Scabies is successfully treated overnight with one application of 5% permethrin cream. Treatment of all the family members should take place at the same time. Clothing and bed sheets should be laundered in hot water and drapes and other items can be placed in plastic bags for 7–10 days. Emollients and antipruritic agents are also helpful but may need to be continued for 1 month. Antibiotics are used as needed on lesions with a bacterial superinfection.

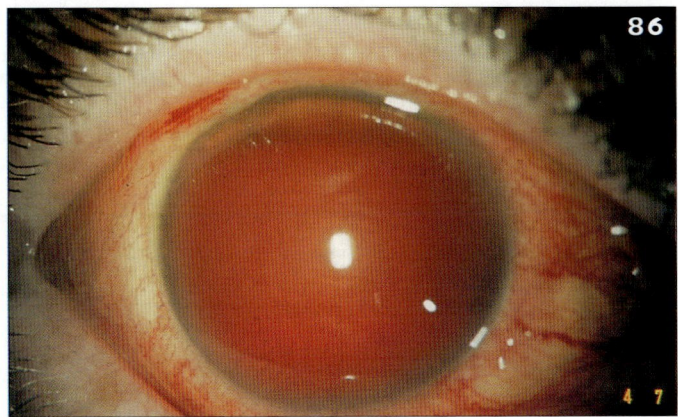

86 What sort of hemorrhages are shown in this fundus (86)?

87 A 1-week-old infant presented with sudden onset of bile stained vomiting. His initial abdominal X-ray is shown (87a).
i. What is the differential diagnosis?
ii. What investigations should be undertaken?
iii. What is the acute management?

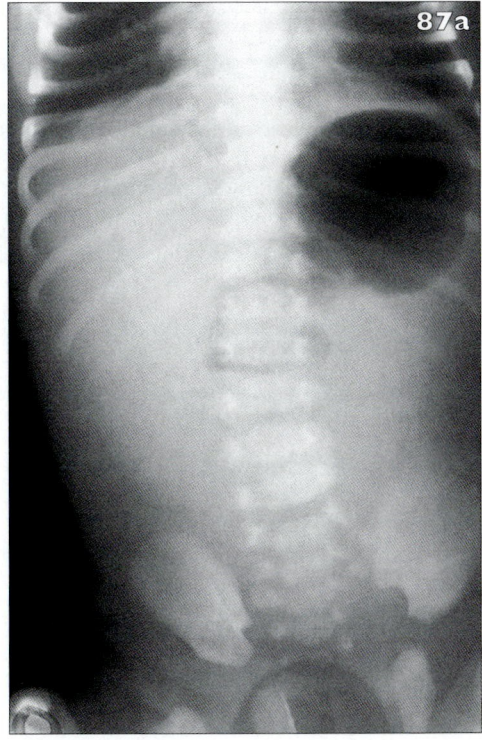

86 The slide shows diffuse vitreous hemorrhage. Anatomically, the vitreous humour is strongly attached to the optic disc margin, the retinal vessels, and the ora serrata of the peripheral retina. Vitreous hemorrhage is secondary to bleeding from retinal blood vessels. It is caused by direct impact rupturing the retinal vessels or indirectly by vitreous traction force on to the retinal vessels. On examination, there is a normal pupillary reaction to light but the red reflex is lost when examined by direct ophthalmoscopy.

Observation is necessary to screen for underlying retinal detachment or retinal tears caused by tractional force of the vitreous base at the ora serrata.

87 i. The diagnosis to exclude is malrotation with volvulus. These children have bile stained vomiting usually with constant abdominal pain. Passage of blood in the stools may occur if ischemia of the bowel has developed.

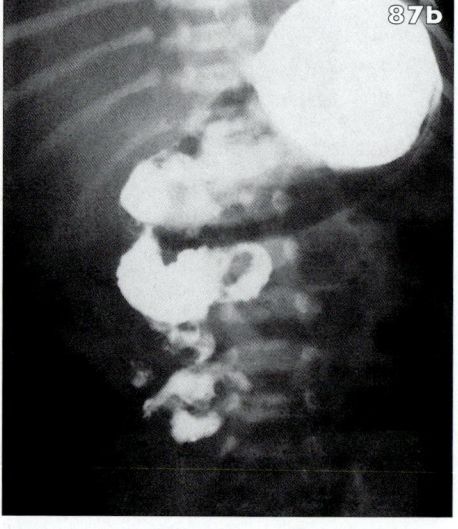

Other diagnoses to consider are: obstruction of the bowel from other causes, e.g. intussusception (rare in this age group), a band across the jejunum, and duplex systems; sepsis, in particular urinary tract infections; and metabolic disorders but these can also present with nonbile stained vomiting.
ii. Investigations include a plain abdominal X-ray (erect and supine) which should be followed by a contrast upper gastrointestinal series in all children with bile stained vomiting to exclude malrotation. This will show a coiled spring appearance of the jejunum (**87b**).
iii. Acute management consists of fluid resuscitation of 10–20 ml/kg of intravenous saline or colloid solution, repeated as necessary. Broad spectrum antibiotics should be given to cover bowel perforation. Urgent surgery is required in a patient with an acute volvulus.

88 This 3-year-old child will only drink milk and eats solid food only sporadically (**88**). Objectively, she is pale, but this is even more pronounced when compared to her mother's skin color. She is playful but slightly less active than she was 1 month ago, and her heart rate is 100 beats/minute at rest.

i. Given the history, physical findings and vital signs, what is the most likely diagnosis?

ii. What abnormalities will be evident on a full blood count which can help confirm the diagnosis?

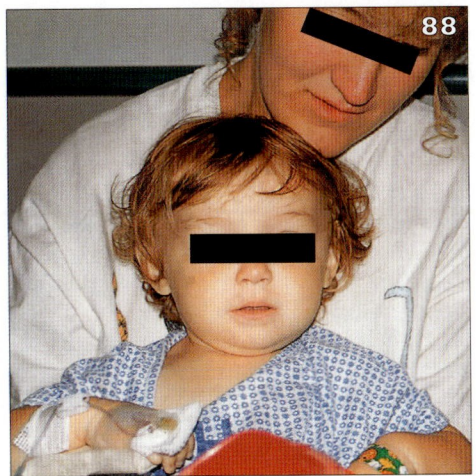

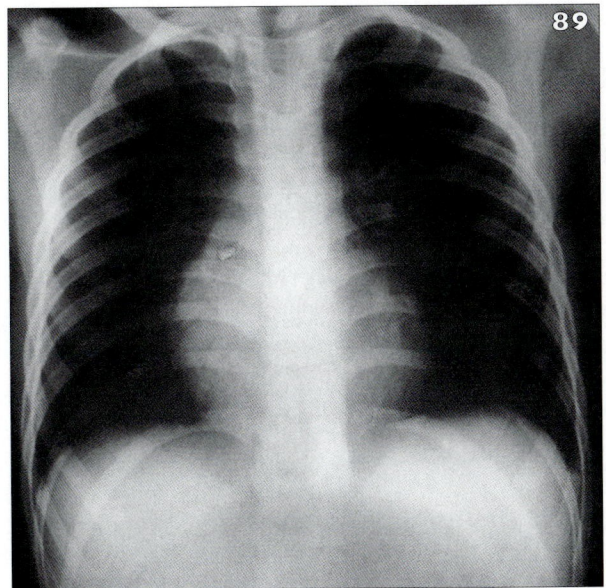

89 A young man fell off some rocks and fractured his femur. Examination revealed that he had lost a tooth during the accident. A pre-anesthetic chest X-ray is shown (**89**).

i. Where is the tooth?

ii. How would you have investigated this child if the foreign body which he was suspected of inhaling had not been radio-opaque?

88 i. The most likely diagnosis is iron deficiency anemia. Her well appearance and normal heart rate suggest that her anemia occurred over an extended period of time. In young children, only 10% of the iron in cow's milk is absorbed, compared to 50% in breast milk. Some children also tend to drink milk preferentially to other iron containing foods.

ii. Aside from a low hemoglobin and hematocrit (this girl's were 38.0 g/l (3.8 g/dl) and 12% respectively), the patient with iron deficiency anemia is expected to have a low mean corpuscular volume, and a high red cell distribution width representing two different populations of cell maturity. A red cell distribution width of >20 is seen commonly in moderate to severe iron deficiency. In addition an increased whole blood protoporphyrin (>35.0 µg/dl (>0.62 µmol/l)) and low serum ferritin (<10.0 µg/l (<1.0 µg/dl)) help to secure the diagnosis.

89 i. The chest X-ray reveals a tooth in the right main bronchus.

ii. Children often present to the emergency department if their parents suspect that they may have inhaled a foreign body with a history of choking and coughing. The children have usually ingested the object rather than inhaled it. However, the potential long term pulmonary consequences of inhaling an object are so serious that once the suspicion of inhalation has been raised, it has to be thoroughly investigated and excluded. Organic objects such as peanuts are particularly damaging as they cause irritation and tissue reaction.

A detailed history of the incident must be taken, noting particularly any abnormalities in swallowing, speaking, or breathing. This must be followed by a thorough examination, especially of the child's mouth, throat, and chest. A normal examination, however, does not exclude inhalation. A generous chest X-ray including the neck, chest, and upper abdomen will show a radio-opaque foreign body in the larynx, trachea, bronchi, esophagus, or stomach and the appropriate management can be instituted. Theoretically, inspiratory and expiratory chest X-rays should show areas of air trapping or collapse, but young children can rarely cooperate with this.

After all the investigations, in some children the situation may still be unclear. Bronchoscopy must therefore be carried out in these cases either to finally exclude the inhalation of a foreign body or remove it if it is present.

90 i. Describe the radiological abnormality shown (**90**), and give the likely diagnosis.
ii. How and at what age does this usually present? What are the usual sites?
iii. What action should you take?

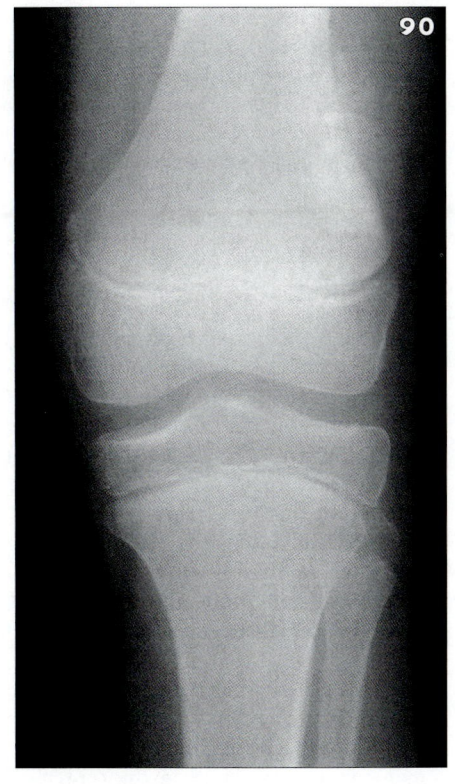

91 A 4-year-old black child presented with vaginal bleeding.
i. What diagnosis does the physical examination suggest (**91**)?
ii. What is the therapy for this condition?

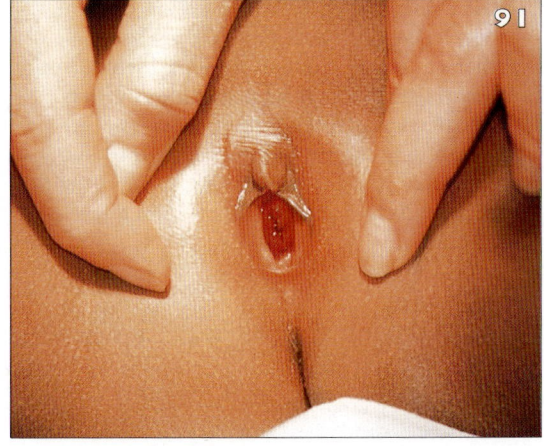

90 i. The X-ray shows a skeletally immature knee with a lesion in the lateral aspect of the distal femoral metaphysis. There is early cortical bone destruction and an adjacent area of irregular, poorly defined calcification extending into the soft tissues.

This is an osteosarcoma. A more dramatic X-ray could have been selected to illustrate the condition but it is important to recognize the more subtle features of a malignant lesion at first presentation because earlier diagnosis allows less mutilating surgery and improved survival.

ii. Osteosarcoma is most common in the second decade and usually occurs in the metaphysis adjacent to rapidly growing physes (distal femur, proximal tibia, and proximal humerus).

The condition most often presents with an asymptomatic swelling or with a dull gnawing pain which has a nonmechanical quality (i.e. present day and night, at rest, and on activity). Occasionally it presents as a pathological fracture through the weakened bone.

iii. Although the exact diagnosis cannot be made from this X-ray there is enough information from the age of the patient, the site of the lesion, and the quality of the lesion to seek urgent radiological advice and referral to an orthopedic surgeon on the presumption that this lesion is an osteosarcoma. The next step ought to be to biopsy the tumor and stage it if the diagnosis is confirmed. This is followed by definitive surgery which may involve amputation or in more favourable cases excision with limb salvage using bone allografts or metallic implants. With adjuvant chemotherapy survival in specialist centers is now over 50%.

91 i. This girl has bleeding caused by local irritation of the urethral mucosa that has prolapsed through its meatus. The physical examination reveals a swollen, well defined, dark red doughnut-shaped tissue covering the vaginal introitus. The urethral lumen can be visualized in the center of this mass. Urethral prolapse is a common cause of vaginal bleeding in black girls between 3–10 years old and is thought to be a result of poor attachment of the smooth muscle layers of the urethra. It can also present with dysuria or even retention of urine. Constipation may also be present and may exacerbate prolapse through straining.

Other causes of vaginal bleeding include trauma, foreign body, vaginitis or from hormonal causes including precocious puberty.

ii. In urethral prolapse, if the mucosa appears healthy and not necrotic, the child can be treated expectantly with saline baths. Many will resolve within a few weeks and will not recur. On the other hand, those patients with obvious necrotic tissue or those whose symptoms do not resolve within a few weeks may require surgical repair.

92 A 3-year-old child was knocked down crossing the road and brought into the emergency department by ambulance. After clinical assessment a chest X-ray was taken (**92**). What do you see?

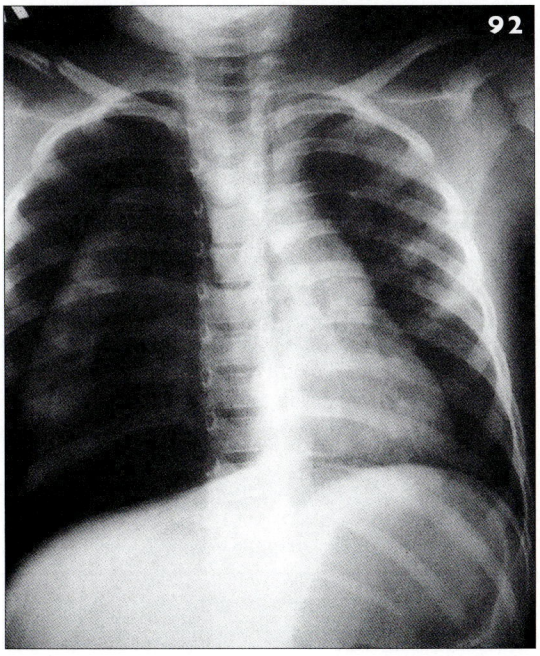

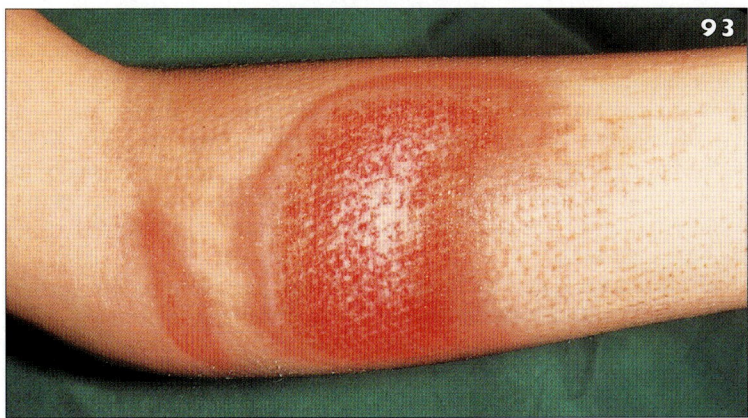

93 This boy caught his forearm in the heavy rollers of his grandmother's wringer (**93**).
i. What superficial injury do you notice?
ii. What other problems must you anticipate, assess, and manage?

92 Three important signs in **92** are:

- The mediastinum is displaced to the left.
- The right lung can be seen surrounded by air.
- The right diaphragm is inverted.

These are the signs of a tension pneumothorax on the right.

Note the clavicular fracture. Fractures of the clavicle and ribs are usually associated with severe trauma. There may be coexistent injury to the vessels in the mediastinum or associated spinal fractures.

It is unusual to see a pneumothorax on a chest film with current trauma protocols. Normally, a symptomatic pneumothorax in a trauma patient is treated following clinical assessment (reduced air entry on the right side, increased percussion note, and mediastinal displacement to the left). An X-ray is taken after placement of the chest drain to see how much of a residual pneumothorax remains. Unnecessary delay waiting for a chest film to be taken may adversely affect clinical management.

93 i. This is a wringer crush injury. This is not so common as it once was but it does illustrate the problems of many crush injuries.

The rollers of the wringer give a crush effect as the arm goes through and then a shearing effect as the arm stops but the rollers continue to turn. This results in deep skin abrasions occasionally with full thickness skin loss requiring skin grafting. In addition, the shearing of subcutaneous tissues can create a large dead space into which bleeding can cause a large hematoma.

ii. The fascial layers around the muscles are usually intact after this injury. However, the crush can cause the muscles to swell massively within the fascia. This can cause pressure within the compartment to rise, reducing capillary blood perfusion below that necessary for tissue viability. This leads to ischemic necrosis and subsequent contractures as muscles are replaced by fibrous tissue.

The clinical signs and symptoms of this compartment syndrome are swelling and tenderness of the affected area with deep persistent aching exacerbated by passive stretching of the muscles, paresis, and paresthesia. The pulses are usually present as the compartmental pressure rarely exceeds central arterial pressure. Compartmental pressure measurement, e.g. use of a needle manometer, is needed to make the definitive measurement.

Treatment must be aimed at improving tissue perfusion in the compartment. Management starts with hospitalization and rest with the arm elevated and regularly observed. However, gross elevation is contraindicated as this lowers tissue perfusion. The patient must be well hydrated. Serum potassium, urea and electrolytes, and urine myoglobin must be monitored. Fasciotomy may be needed to relieve the pressure but it must be adequate and must decompress the whole compartment.

X-rays are often taken in these sort of injuries but fractures are rarely found.

94 A 13-year-old has left sided scrotal pain and vomiting, which developed suddenly when he was out biking with his friends. His scrotal area is shown (**94**).
i. What are the most likely diagnoses?
ii. What physical findings are important in determining the diagnosis and outcome for this patient?

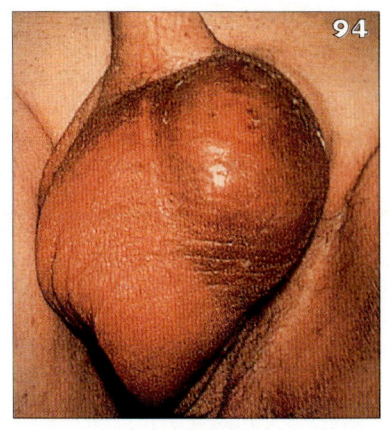

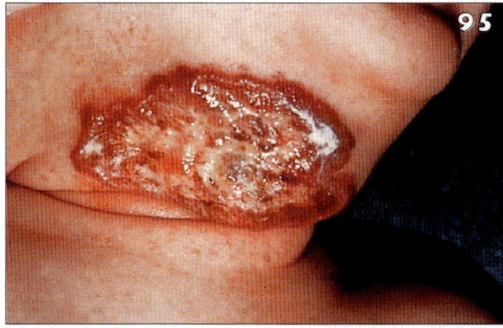
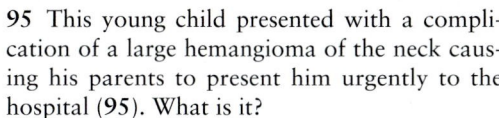

95 This young child presented with a complication of a large hemangioma of the neck causing his parents to present him urgently to the hospital (**95**). What is it?

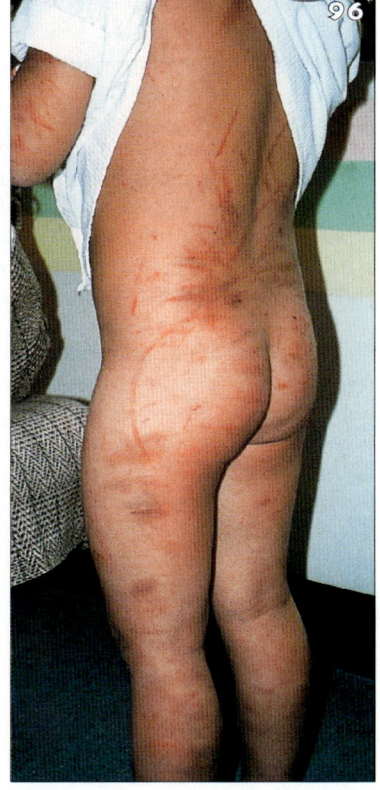

96 A 3-year-old child is brought to the emergency department by the police after being found alone in her home. You identify numerous patterned bruises on her body during your examination (**96**). The remainder of the examination is normal, including a neurological examination. How would you complete your medical assessment?

94 i. The most likely diagnosis for this patient is testicular torsion or epididymitis. Given the discoloration of the left scrotal sac, it is likely that he has torsion of the spermatic cord causing congestion and swelling. Torsion of the testis is most common in the neonatal period and around puberty. In the latter group it may present as lower abdominal pain or groin pain. It may have an acute or gradual onset. Intermittent torsion gives a diagnostic dilemma.

ii. The presence of a brisk cremasteric reflex would argue strongly against the diagnosis of testicular torsion, with a negative predictive value of over 90%. The length of time lapsed between onset of pain and eventual detorsion is the most important factor in determining the viability of the affected testis. Viability of the torsed testis 24 hours after symptom onset is rare.

Other investigations such as Doppler ultrasonography are being developed as a tool to diagnose the torsion by indicating testicular blood flow. However, no matter how sensitive the test is, if it relies on perfusion it will only indicate the state of the perfusion at the time of the test. It will not exclude previous or future torsion.

95 The lesion shows partial ulceration. This only affects a minority of hemangiomas and is most likely to occur during the period of rapid growth of the lesion in the first year of life. Hemangiomas of the perineal area are especially at risk of this complication. Secondary infection and bleeding can also occur, most commonly involving lesions of the lips, mouth, and anogenital regions. Careful hygiene, topical and systemic antibiotics, and dressings may be needed to minimize cellulitis and scarring. The bleeding is distressing for the parents but can easily be controlled by direct pressure. Occasionally ulcerating hemangiomas respond to pulsed dye laser treatment.

Hemangiomas of the head and neck can be associated with subglottic hemangiomas presenting as airway obstruction. Complications of large hemangiomas include thrombocytopenia, caused by platelet trapping within the lesion (Kasabach–Merritt syndrome) and high output cardiac failure. Prednisolone orally can be effective in these situations.

96 The distribution, multiplicity, and pattern of the marks are diagnostic of inflicted trauma. An evaluation for bleeding diathesis is recommended to exclude a bleeding disorder. Some physicians would consider completing a skeletal survey to evaluate for occult bony injury. In general, skeletal surveys have a low yield in children over 2 years old, and in such children should be completed only if there is a reason to suspect skeletal trauma (tenderness, deformity, and severe nonbony injuries). Given the distribution of the marks over the buttocks and thighs a urinalysis is recommended to search for indicators of rhabdomyolysis and myoglobinuria. A positive urine dip for blood, without red blood cells suggests the diagnosis. This can most easily be confirmed with a serum creatinine phosphokinase level. Because some physically injured children may have occult abdominal trauma, serum liver function, and pancreatic tests are recommended. Finally, do not forget your legal mandate to report the abuse to the local authorities for further investigation.

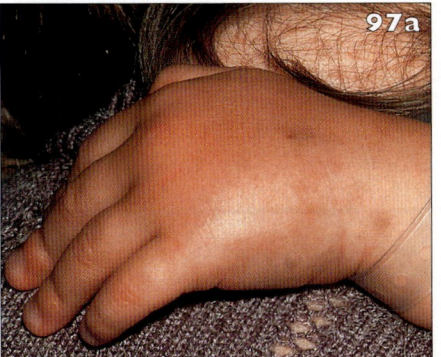

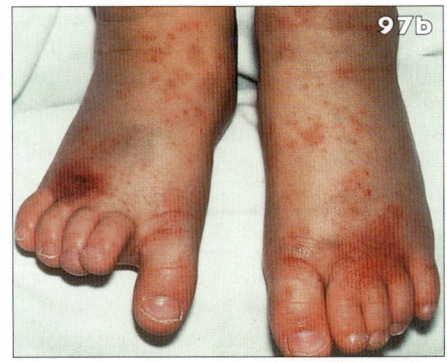

97 This 3-year-old boy presented with puffiness around the eyes and on the dorsum of both hands, together with raised purpuric rash affecting mainly the extensor aspects of the limbs and buttocks (**97a–c**).
i. What is the likely diagnosis?
ii. What is the management?
iii. What information should be imparted to the parents?

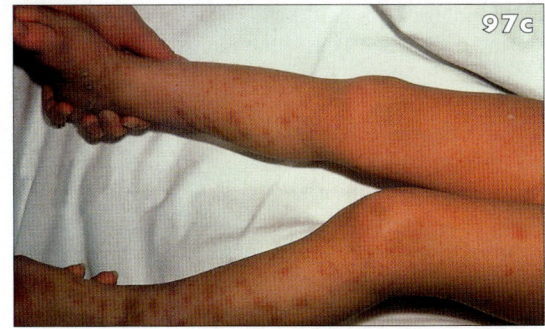

98 This 6-year-old girl presented with a firm, nontender 3 × 2 cm (1 × 0.75 in) swelling in the right side of the neck (**98**). The swelling had been present for several weeks, but had recently become larger with redness of the overlying skin. She was a keen swimmer.
i. What is the differential diagnosis?
ii. What are the initial investigations?

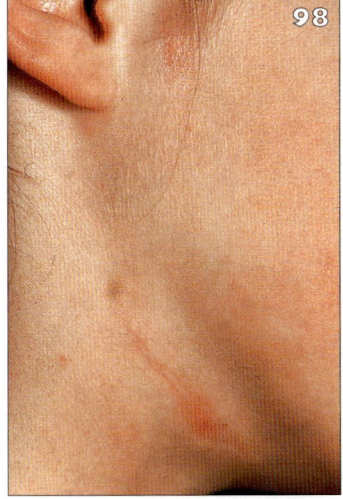

97 i. Henoch–Schönlein (anaphylactoid) purpura.

ii. No specific therapy is available. If hemolytic streptococci are detected (in around 20% of cases) penicillin is indicated. Rest should be encouraged during the acute phase as physical activity tends to exacerbate the rash and the joint involvement. Symptomatic treatment is helpful. The only indication for steroid treatment is severe and intractable abdominal pain.

iii. The condition is common in young children, often follows a mild viral infection, and in most children clears up completely. It may come and go and come again before clearing fully. The usual duration is up to 6 weeks but can be as long as a year or more. The kidneys and gut may also be involved in the generalized 'allergic' condition. Urine and blood pressure therefore need to be checked for a while.

The joints – especially the weight bearing ones – often become transiently swollen.

If the illness occurs in the summer months, insect repellents should be used when the child goes out of doors, as hypersensitivity reactions around bites may be marked during the early phase of the illness.

98 i. This child has chronic unilateral cervical lymphadenitis. As the swelling is not painful nor tender, it is most likely to have been caused by *Mycobacterium tuberculosis* or atypical mycobacterial infection (e.g. *M. avium intracellulare*). It is important to enquire about BCG immunization and contact with tuberculosis. The most common cause of this appearance is infection with *M. avium* or *M. scrofulaceum*. However, this girl is a keen swimmer and may have been infected with *M. marinum* from a swimming pool.

Other possible causes of this appearance include: cervical pyogenic abscess, glandular fever, and malignancy.

ii. The initial investigations include Mantoux test, chest X-ray, monospot test, Epstein–B virus antibodies, full blood count, blood film, ESR, and throat swab.

Superficial lymph node involvement in tuberculosis commonly affects cervical or supraclavicular nodes, secondary to a focus in the tonsils or upper respiratory tract.

In atypical infection, the treatment of choice is by total excision of the node(s) involved. Chemotherapy is likely to be ineffective.

99 This 9-month-old baby presents with a rash that has been present for 3 weeks (**99**). His mother has been using saline baths and topical over-the-counter ointment.
i. What is your diagnosis?
ii. What treatment do you recommend?

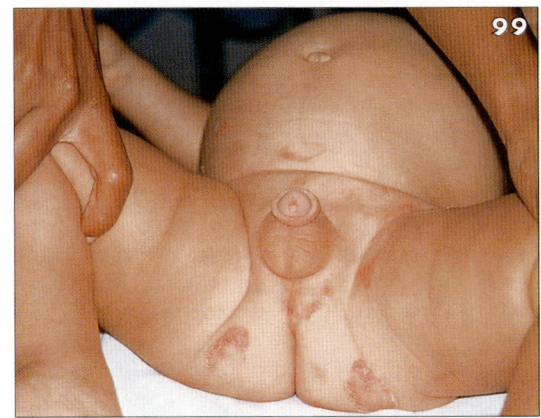

100 A 14-year-old boy saw the primary care provider on three occasions over the previous 6 weeks because of left knee pain. He then attended the local emergency department where examination and X-rays of the knee were normal. The emergency department physician asked for advice from an orthopedic surgeon. After observing the boy lying on the couch, he requested hip X-rays (**100a, b**).
i. What does he think is wrong?
ii. At what age does this usually present?

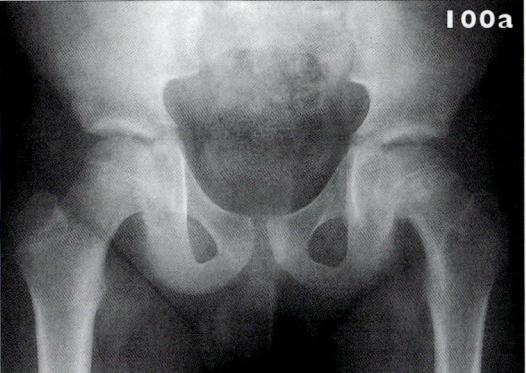

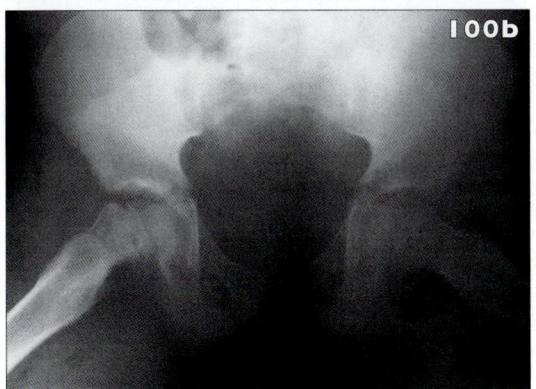

99 i. This patient has impetigo, an infection of the superficial epidermis. The rash usually begins on skin already damaged, for instance by an abrasion or an insect bite with red macules that develop into thin roofed vesicles on an erythematous base. As these lesions rupture, a honey colored fluid is released. Over half of cases are due to *Staphylococcus aureus* infection, and the remaining to group A streptococcal infection. Complications of cellulitis and disseminated disease can occur.

ii. Swabs should be taken to confirm the organism and the sensitivities and treatment should be started while awaiting the results. Topical antibiotics such as mupirocin or bacitracin ointments are effective. With extensive skin involvement, oral antibiotics such as flucloxacillin or erythromycin effective against both organisms may be added. Patients must have separate face cloths, towels, and bed sheets from the rest of the family.

The sensitivity of organisms changes with locality and time. Antibiotic prescribing must therefore be undertaken with knowledge of the local resistance.

100 i. This patient has a slipped upper (or capital) femoral epiphysis (SUFE or SCFE). Hip pathology is relatively common in children, ranging from congenital hip dislocation in infants through transient synovitis and Perthe's disease later in childhood to SUFE which occurs most often, but not exclusively in adolescents.

ii. The cause of SUFE is unknown in most cases but rarely it is associated with endocrine abnormalities such as hypothyroidism or with renal osteodystrophy which is thought to weaken the growth plate. It occurs most often at the growth spurt (11–13 years in girls and 12–14 years in boys) and in overweight individuals suggesting that the active growth plate is relatively weak in supporting the increased bodyweight.

The clinical presentation is usually of a susceptible individual with hip discomfort, which may be very mild, and a limp or of a susceptible individual with knee pain only. The importance of recognizing referred pain from hip to knee cannot be over-emphasized.

The X-rays show a minor but definite abnormality of the left hip with the capital epiphysis slipping downwards and backwards off the metaphysis (compared to the opposite side). The lateral view (the so-called frog lateral view) usually shows the slip more clearly and because the femoral neck has slid anteriorly relative to the epiphysis the leg lies in external rotation and it is now clearer why the orthopedic consultant requested the hip X-rays on seeing the leg posture.

At first it seems surprising that little discomfort is felt in the presence of what could be considered a growth plate fracture (Salter–Harris type 1), but then it is important to realize that the slip is glacial in its speed because the epiphysis is not separated but rather it is weakly fixed. When pathological events occur slowly the presentation is seldom dramatic.

101 Should the child in **100** be treated as an emergency, urgently, or routinely?

102 A 6-year-old child complains of pain in the peri-rectal area shown (**102**). What is the diagnosis and what is the etiology?

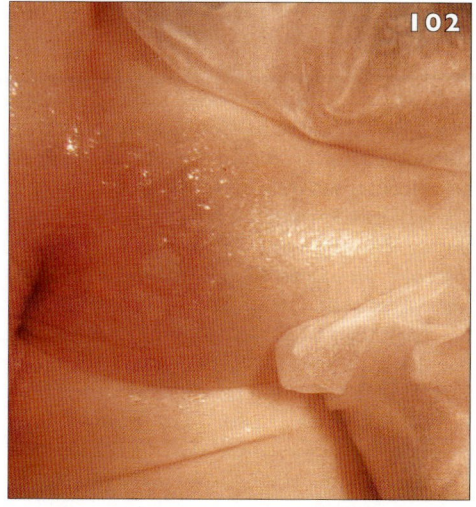

103 A 7-year-old child presented with a persistent cough, fever, and weight loss despite treatment from his primary care provider.
i. What do you see on the chest X-ray (**103**)?
ii. What other tests might support your diagnosis?

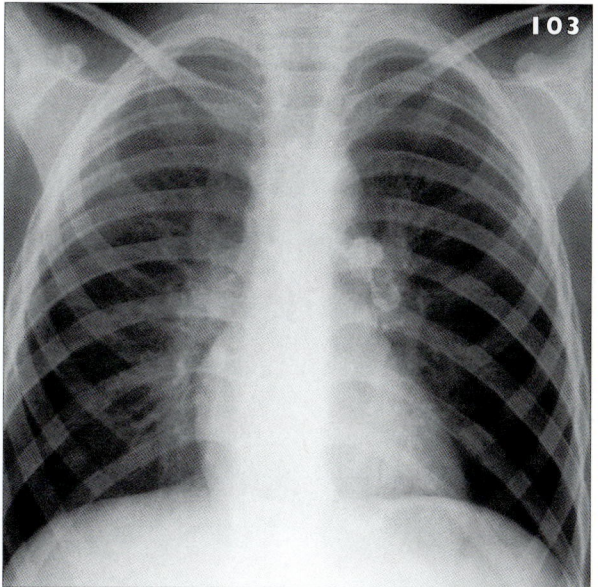

101 This patient should be treated urgently, that is admitted from the emergency department for bedrest pending screw fixation of the epiphysis on the next day's operating list. Untreated the epiphysis slips further and further off the femoral neck creating more deformity and posing technical difficulties passing screws. About 30% of patients go on to have similar problems with the other side and some surgeons prophylactically fix the other epiphysis at the same time.

102 The findings are vesicular lesions of peri-rectal herpes infection. Anogenital lesions were thought to be predominantly caused by herpesvirus type 2 and spread by sexual contact. However, recent surveys of the infection have shown almost equal numbers of infection caused by type 1 and type 2.

The virus is passed by close personal contact and in the neonate from the mother during delivery, when the presenting part, head or bottom, is the most common site of infection. In older children, the cause may be genital to genital contact or orogenital or anogenital contact. However, a case has been reported from a recurrent herpetic whitlow on a mother's hand and autoinoculation could occur, for example from the child's own herpetic whitlow. It is noteworthy that adults who have no history of herpes infection and those in remission from their recurrent condition can both shed viruses.

The gold standard for identification is by virus culture from vesicular fluid taken from the base of a vesicle. The recent development of restriction enzyme technology has allowed 'finger printing' of strains and has been used to show the uniqueness of strains from an individual. If isolates from a child thought to have been abused matched those from a suspected perpetrator, this would be strong evidence of sexual abuse.

In this case, when interviewed, this child reported sexual contact with an adult family member. In such cases, local child protection procedures must be initiated to ensure the safety of the child.

103 i. The heart size is normal and the lungs are clear. There is calcification in nodes of the left hilum. The most common cause for this appearance is tuberculosis.

The diagnosis is a healed Ghon focus. The peripheral lung lesion giving rise to the calcified regional glands may not be visible on radiography. The clinical history suggests reactivation of tuberculosis, although the lungs appear radiographically clear.
ii. Children with active tuberculosis might show a high ESR and C-reactive protein. A Mantoux test shows an induration of more than 5 mm (0.2 in) and sputum or early morning stomach aspirate may be positive for acid-fast bacilli.

104 This boy was bitten while playing with his aunt's cat earlier in the day (**104**). He now complains of pain in his hand.
i. What is your diagnosis?
ii. What is the appropriate treatment?

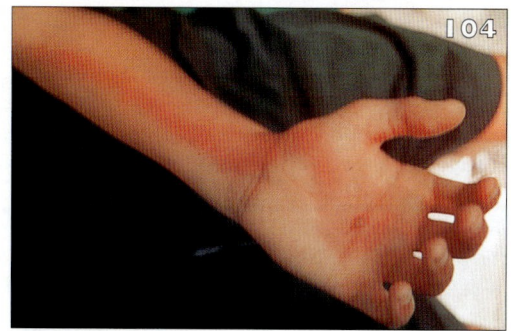

105 A 7-year-old girl came to the emergency department with an acutely painful and discharging ear. This was the appearance down the auroscope (**105**). What is your diagnosis and how should you treat it?

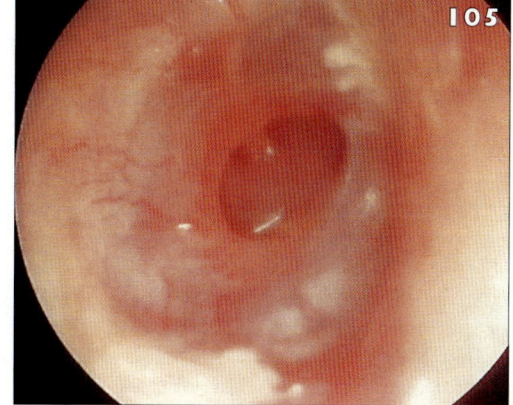

106 This small boy, too young to give a history, was said to have burned his hand on the front of a cooker (**106**).
i. What is the likely mechanism of injury of this lesion?
ii. What measures would you take to manage this case in addition to the simple treatment for the injury?

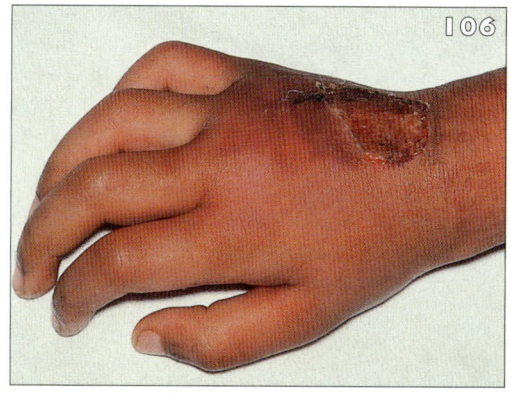

104 i. This boy has cellulitis resulting from a cat bite. Dog bites are the most common sort of animal bites in children, but a significant number of children are bitten by cats. Cats do not usually cause as much tissue damage as dogs. If left untreated 50% of cat bites will become infected with *Pasteurella multocida*. Other bacteria found in infected cat bites are *Staphylococcus*, *Streptococcus*, and *Bacteroides* species. Rarely cat bites can also transmit cat scratch fever, Q fever, and toxoplasmosis.

ii. Good wound management is the basis of management of animal bites. Treatment of cat bites that are not yet infected involves copious irrigation and debridement. If bleeding is controlled and cosmetic appearance is not a consideration, the puncture wounds or lacerations should not be sutured closed. Cosmetically significant wounds of the face or scalp can be closed after wound toilet as they have a good blood supply but must be carefully observed for infection which will usually become apparent after 24 hours.

Prophylactic oral antibiotics should be prescribed in all but the most superficial wounds, and in wounds in elderly and immunocompromized patients. Co-amoxiclav or erythromycin and metronidazole are suitable antibiotics. Tetanus prophylaxis should be given in unimmunized patients and rabies prophylaxis should be considered. It is very rare, however, in domestic animals in Western Europe and North America. Once an infection has developed, as in this case, intravenous antibiotics are indicated.

105 A large central perforation of the tympanic membrane is shown. The middle ear is acutely inflamed and moist. She has an acute on chronic otitis media.

The management should include sending a swab for culture to the laboratory, gently mopping the pus out of the ear, and the use of antibiotics such as amoxicillin. In certain locations, 25% of *Haemophilus influenzae* infections are resistant to amoxicillin. Local sensitivities must be borne in mind when choosing an antibiotic. The use of antibiotic ear drops may help resolution if it is slow to clear. Once the ear has settled there may be a place for repair of the tympanic membrane (myringoplasty).

Otitis media should be part of the differential diagnosis of a child with unexplained fever. There is no ear pain in 20% of cases of otitis media and there is wax covering the ear drum in many cases. The wax should be removed to allow better examination of the ear drum.

106 i. This child has sustained a contact burn to his hand. The normal behavior and development of a child must be taken into account when one is assessing an injury to a child. Small children explore the world with the palm of the hand, not the dorsum. Accidental contact burns from hot cooker fronts are therefore overwhelmingly likely to be on the palm. This injury is highly unlikely to have been accidental.

ii. A child protection investigation was initiated. This injury proved to be non-accidental and on further social work and police investigation further concerns about the care of the child were uncovered. The child was taken into care for his own safety.

107 This 4-year-old girl presented to the emergency department with a 2 week history of easy bruising (**107**), and was thought to have idiopathic thrombocytopenic purpura.

i. What other conditions should be considered in the differential diagnosis?

ii. What initial investigations are required?

iii. What treatments are available?

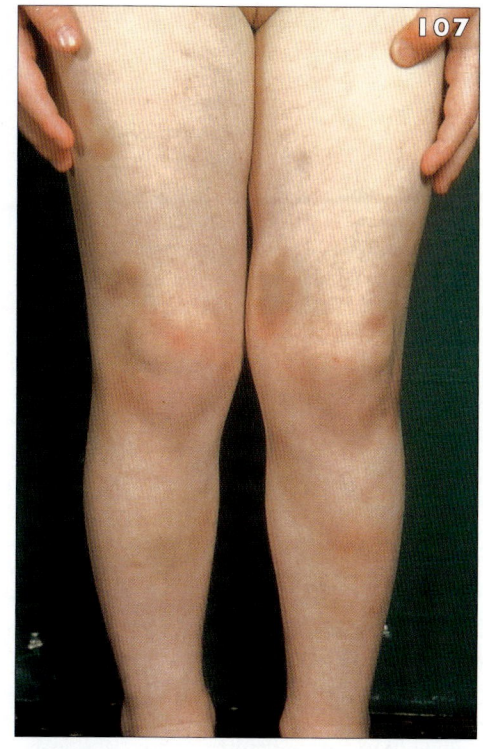

108 A child has presented to the emergency department with difficulty in breathing and a progressive loss of voice over the preceding month. A view of the larynx when the child was in theatre is shown (**108**).

i. What is your diagnosis?

ii. What is the cause of the condition and what is the usual treatment?

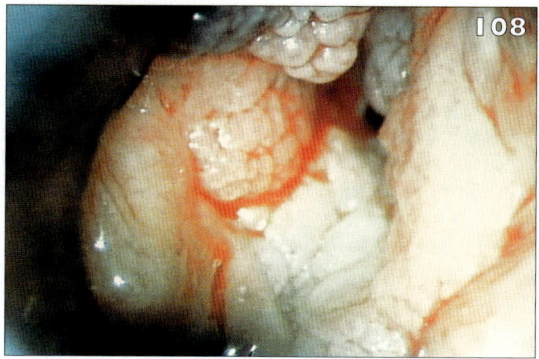

107 i. Other conditions include: leukemia, thrombocytopenia/absent radii, Henoch–Schönlein purpura, nonaccidental injury, and coagulation disorders.

ii. A full blood count with platelet count and a film is needed.

In the presence of thrombocytopenia there is no significant excess of bleeding with mild trauma until the platelet count falls below $50–60 \times 10^9/l$ ($50–60 \times 10^3/mm^3$). Spontaneous bruising rarely occurs when the platelet count is above $20 \times 10^9/l$ ($20 \times 10^3/mm^3$). Coagulation tests are normal but the bleeding time is prolonged.

Examination of the bone marrow must be the next step if treatment with steroids is contemplated as other conditions such as leukemia and aplastic anemia may mimic idiopathic thrombocytopenic purpura.

iii. This child has idiopathic thrombocytopenic purpura, a disease which usually remits spontaneously and completely. However, in about 10% of cases remission is not sustained. So long as the platelet count does not fall too low, bringing the risk of intracranial hemorrhage, no treatment is necessary.

Where treatment is needed approximately 50% of patients respond to an initial course of steroids, although the platelets can fall again when the steroids are tapered off. If further treatment is needed gammaglobulin or anti-D globulin usually gives a temporary increase in the platelet count. Immunosuppressive therapy such as vincristine rarely works and splenectomy should only very rarely be used.

108 i. This child has laryngeal papillomatosis almost occluding the airway. The chest was almost silent on auscultation. There was no stridor because of the soft nature of the airway obstruction but there was no voice.

ii. The condition is caused by the human papilloma virus and may present at any age but usually in infancy. It is more common in first born children who are delivered vaginally in teenage mothers. Boys and girls are equally affected. The papillomata may appear at other sites in the respiratory and digestive tracts, e.g. the trachea and bronchi and lesions can sometimes be seen on examination of the nasal or oral cavities.

In a case so severe as this, the management is immediate treatment to remove the papillomata, usually by laser under general anesthetic. The condition is recurrent and repeated procedures throughout childhood may be required for control of the airway, although most children ultimately enter spontaneous remission usually by puberty. Malignant change can occur in the papillomata in children, but is very rare and usually occurs in the tracheopulmonary tree rather than the larynx.

Adult onset papillomatosis is a sexually transmitted disease.

109 A 13-year-old basketball player 'jammed' his finger while getting a rebound ball (**109**).
i. What is his injury?
ii. How should you treat it?

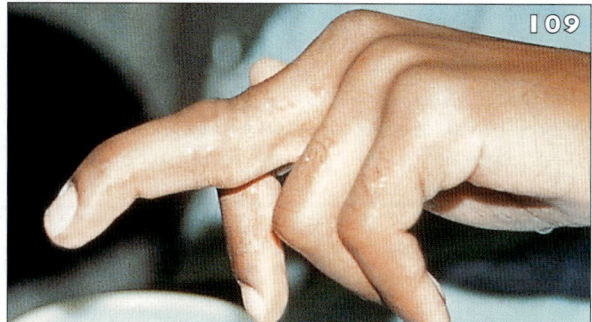

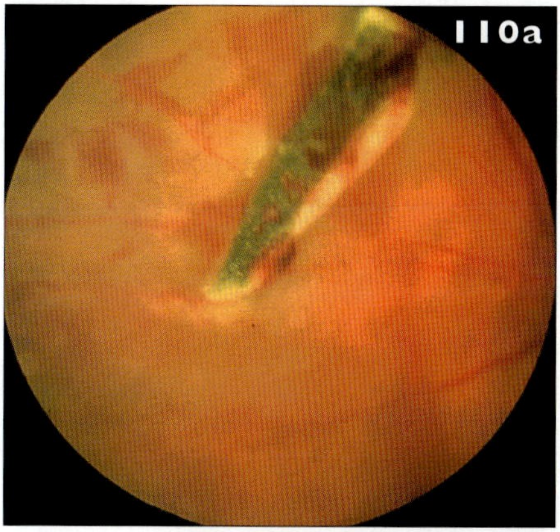

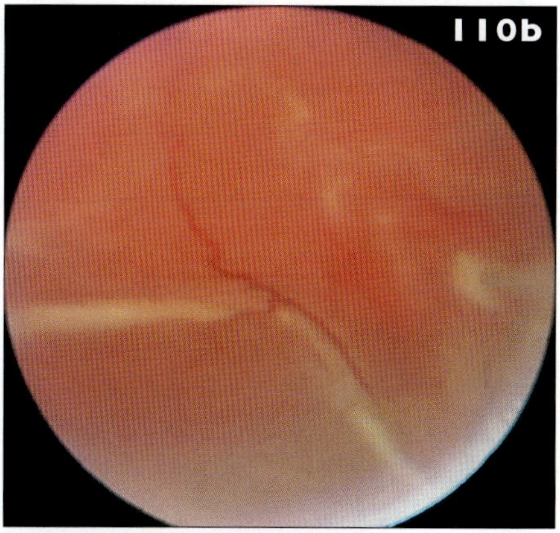

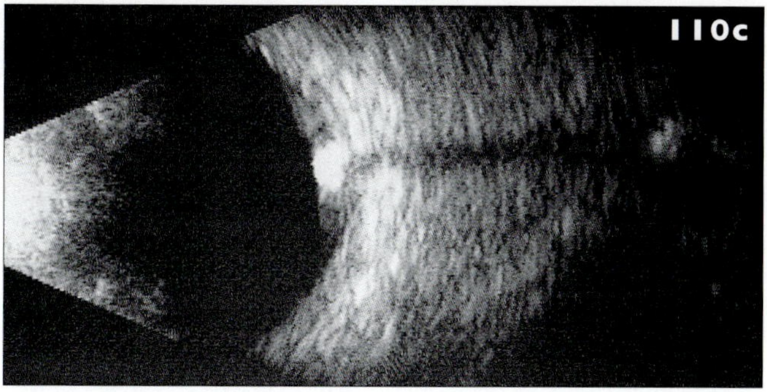

110 Three perforating eye injuries caused by foreign bodies are shown (**110a–c**).
i. Where is the foreign body in each case?
ii. What would be your immediate medical management and investigation?

109 i. Joint dislocations are common sports related injuries, usually resulting from an axial compression by contact with the ball. They usually affect the 'outboard' digits, i.e. the thumb, forefinger, and little finger, although in this case the middle finger is affected. This child had a dislocated proximal interphalangeal joint. Radiographic evaluation of this injury is necessary to identify any associated avulsion fractures indicating injury to the collateral ligaments or tendon insertions.

ii. For treatment, regional anesthesia can be provided in the form of a digital block. Reduction can then be achieved with steady longitudinal/distraction traction. If there is no associated avulsion fracture and there is ligamentous stability after reduction, immobilization with a splint for several days followed by buddy strapping with active movement is indicated. If there is an associated avulsion fracture of greater than one-third of the joint surface or ligamentous instability, then operative treatment and often internal fixation is necessary.

Dislocations which are difficult to reduce may be complicated by button-holing of the head of the bone through the capsule with entrapment of soft tissue.

110 i. 110a A vitreous foreign body with adjacent vitreous and retinal hemorrhage.

110b An area of bullous retinal detachment caused by a retinal hole or tear caused by an intraocular foreign body. Fluid from the vitreous cavity accumulates under the retina and separates it off from the underlying retinal pigment epithelium and choroid.

110c An intraocular foreign body on the retinal surface with a high reflectivity signal detected by echography.

ii. Immediate medical treatment may include systemic appropriate analgesics and anti-emetics and assessment of tetanus status.

If there is a possibility of an intraocular foreign body, skull and orbit radiography is mandatory. Other imaging techniques e.g. CT and ultrasonography may be helpful. Magnetic imaging may be useful for localizing a nonmagnetic metallic foreign body.

All cases of suspected perforating injury or intraocular foreign body require referral to the eye department and the emergency department physician should not attempt to remove any protruding material from the eye before the transfer.

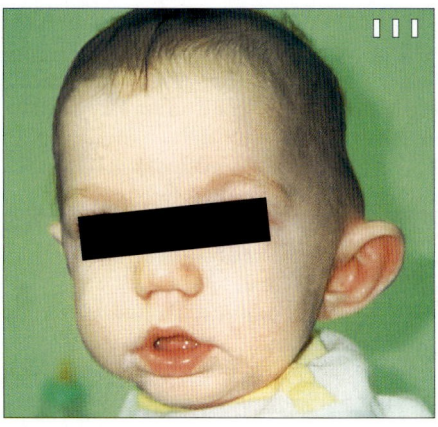

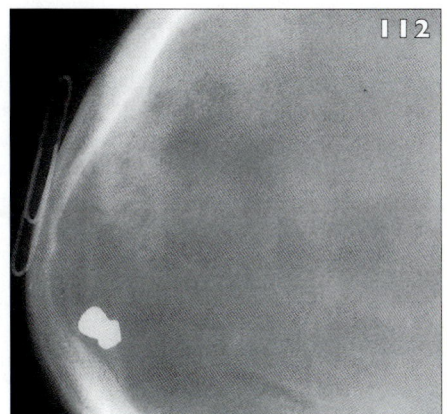

111 This child's parents claim that his ear is protruding more in the last 2 days (**111**).
i. What clinical manifestations might one expect to find in this child's condition?
ii. What are the causative organisms involved in the pathogenesis of this condition?

112 A 6-year-old child was walking to school when he became aware of a sudden pain in his head. A 12-year-old boy was looking out of the window of a second floor room and appeared to be playing with a toy. The emergency department doctor took this X-ray (**112**).
i. What does the X-ray show? What serious clinical problems may arise?
ii. Why is it particularly important to document accurate and detailed recording of the history and examination in such a case?

113 What abnormalities do you see in this child (**113**), and what would be your immediate management?

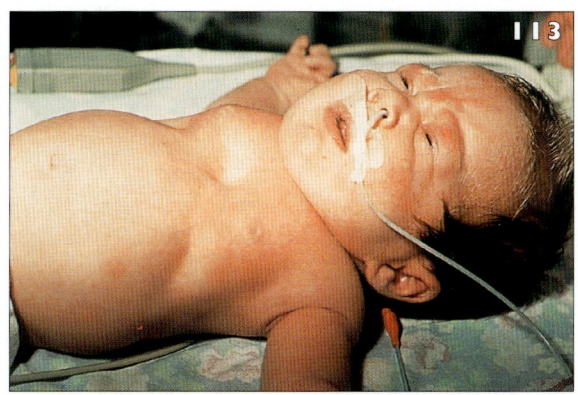

111 i. The child has acute mastoiditis. He would be expected to have a fever of more than 38.3°C (100.9°F), mastoid tenderness and/or erythema, and forward and lateral displacement of the auricle. Displacement of the ear downwards and out is characteristic in children of under 1 year of age. In addition, the child must have a concomitant otitis media in order to secure the diagnosis.

Mastoid X-rays may reveal opacity of the mastoid air cells and there may also be some bone destruction secondary to the osteomyelitis of the surrounding bone.

ii. The most common bacteriological culprits in acute mastoiditis are *Streptococcus* and *Staphylococcus* species, *Klebsiella pneumoniae* and *Pseudomonas aeruginosa*. Chronic mastoiditis is more commonly caused by *Pseudomonas* species.

All children will need admission for intravenous antibiotics. Drainage is only needed if the child is severely ill or if there is intracranial spread of the infection.

112 i. The X-ray shows an opacity suggestive of an air gun pellet in the scalp tissues. It is potentially dangerous as it may result in penetration of vital tissues such as the eye where it could lead to loss of vision.

ii. In such an injury, legal action is often taken by the parent or child. Accurate documentation is important to ensure that the medical evidence is clear and accurate. The emotional effects of the injury on the child should also be noted and documented.

113 This child has severe upper airways obstruction. The child looks anxious. There is flaring of the nostrils, intercostal and sternal recession, and paradoxical movement of the chest and abdomen during respiration. No further examination, in particular of the upper airway or throat should be undertaken.

Whatever the cause of the obstruction, this child is at severe risk and immediate measures need to be taken to support the airway. The child should be admitted without delay to a pediatric intensive care unit and should be assessed by an ENT surgeon with expertise in airway obstruction in infants. The oxygen saturation should be monitored carefully, but no distressing procedures such as venepuncture should be carried out until the staff and equipment to support the airways are to hand. Oxygen should be administered by face mask. Airway support by endotracheal intubation may well be necessary. This child has subglottic stenosis and ultimately underwent emergency tracheostomy. Until the introduction of a vaccine against *Haemophilus influenzae*, epiglottitis was the commonest cause of acute airway obstruction in young children.

114 A child presented with a 2 day history of a limp.
i. What does this pelvis X-ray show (**114**)?
ii. His mother is a nurse in the orthopedic department and can see the X-ray. She is alarmed by these appearances. What do you tell her about the development of these appearances and her child's prognosis?

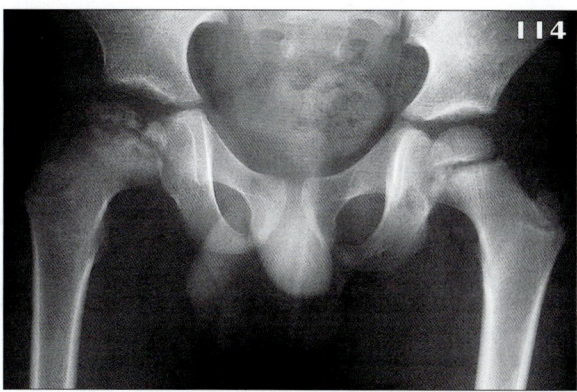

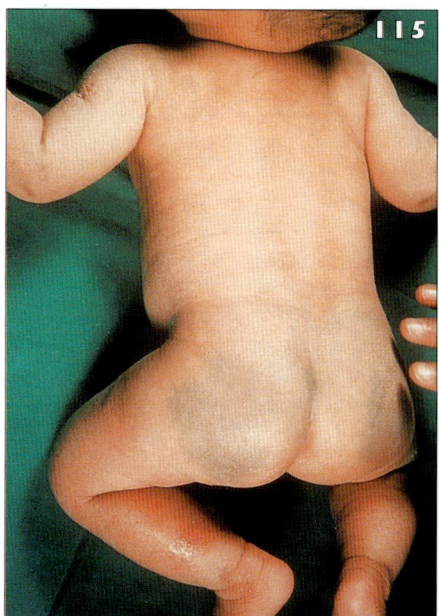

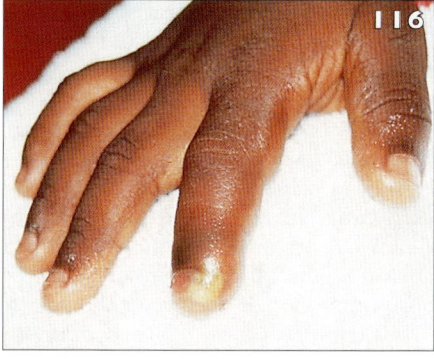

116 This 3-year-old boy has been crying that his finger hurts (**116**). His mother can not recall any injury to that finger.
i. What is your diagnosis?
ii. How would you treat this child?

115 This baby with severe infantile eczema was referred by a health visitor as she was worried about bruising to his bottom (**115**). What is the cause of the lesion? What is the natural history of the condition?

114 i. The X-ray shows right-sided Perthe's disease.

This is best regarded as an idiopathic form of spontaneous avascular necrosis of the femoral head. The child is usually aged between 4 and 8 years, fit and well in himself and presents with either a limp or minor hip or knee pain of several weeks or months duration. However, the presentation is occasionally of similar pain of short duration and relatively sudden onset, even though the X-rays may show long standing changes.
ii. The radiological features depend on the stage at which the child presents but in general terms the femoral head looks dense and collapsed down. Later a mottled appearance develops as old dead bone is removed and new bone is deposited. Finally the cycle is complete (about 2 years) and the child is left with a mushroom shaped femoral head which functions well until middle age when degenerative changes tend to occur. The often dramatic radiographic changes alarm the parents especially when the opposite hip is shown for comparison.

In the initial stages of the disease the child often has clinical symptoms of an irritable hip and in the absence of features suggesting sepsis, rest is all that is required pending an orthopedic out-patient appointment. Occasionally in the long term management splints are provided and surgery is performed to try and improve the shape of the femoral head but indications for any treatment at all are very controversial.

115 This baby of Chinese origin has an extensive blue–black pigmented area at the base of his back and on his buttocks, a so-called 'blue spot'.

An area of pigmentation at this site is a normal finding on the trunk and proximal extremities in pigmented babies. It can also be found occasionally in babies of Caucasian origin. It gradually fades over the first 2–3 years, or is camouflaged by normal pigmentation. There are rarer variants where unilateral patchy dermal melanosis of the skin of the face or shoulder regions persists into adult life.

It is important to recognize this condition. It is extremely distressing to families if it is misdiagnosed as bruising and a child protection investigation is initiated. It is useful, therefore for the mark to be documented in health records as early as possible to be used as a point of reference at later medical examinations.

116 i. He has a paronychia, an infection of the basal or lateral nail fold. It is usually caused by biting of the cuticle or a minor crush injury to the fingertip. It presents as a tender bulge at the nail fold with a central white/yellow area and surrounding erythema. The differential diagnosis of this includes herpetic whitlow and a felon (an infection in the fat pad spaces or volar pulp of the distal phalanx).
ii. If the infection is identified early in the course, it can be treated with a finger cot and antibiotic ointment. These provide a warm, wet environment with gentle maceration of the area to open and drain the infection. If the infection is advanced, an incision with a scalpel followed by warm soaks and oral antibiotics is indicated.

117 A 2-year-old girl was brought to the emergency department after falling with a pencil in her mouth. She was drooling and had dysphagia. What complication is indicated by her lateral neck X-ray (**117**)?

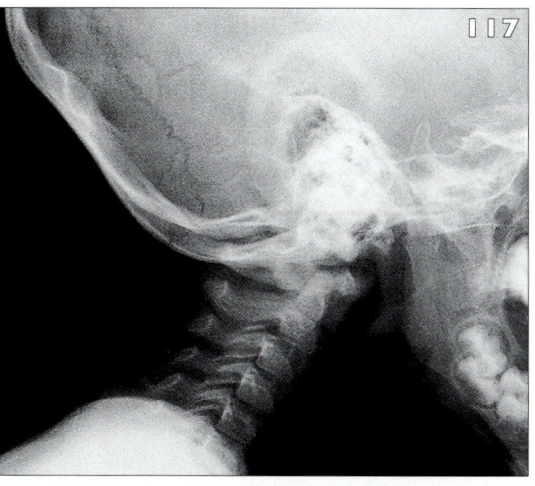

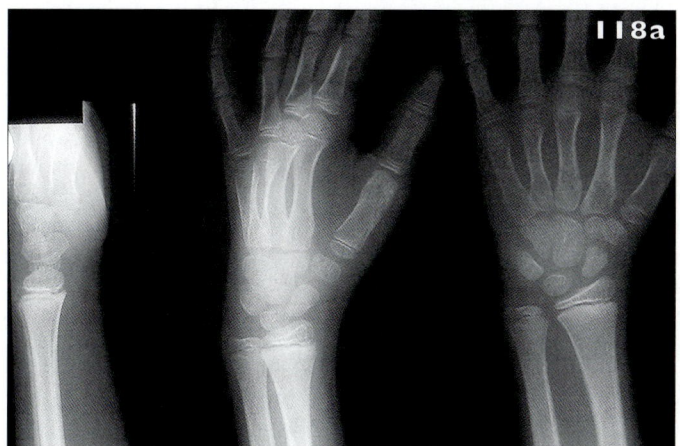

118 A child has fallen on her outstretched hand and has pain around the radial aspect of the wrist.
i. What injury does this X-ray show (**118a**)?
ii. What clinical findings would you expect to find?
iii. What investigation is shown (**118b**)? Why was it undertaken?
iv. What treatment and follow-up is needed?

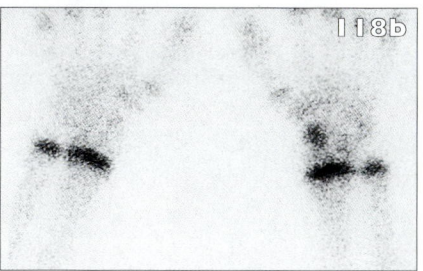

117 The X-ray shows retropharyngeal air from a laceration of the pharyngeal wall. Examination of the neck may show subcutaneous emphysema and a chest X-ray would help to detect air tracking into the mediastinum. Another possible complication is mediastinitis.

118 i. The X-ray shows a normal wrist.
ii. Specifically there was tenderness on palpation in the anatomical snuffbox. These are the features suggestive of a scaphoid fracture exactly as in adults. They are not, however, specific and in the presence of normal X-rays the patient was treated symptomatically using a Colles type below elbow plaster cast. In this case the cast was removed 10–14 days later because the clinical signs persisted. Further X-rays were requested. These were again normal.
iii. An isotope bone scan is shown (**118b**). It was requested to clarify the nature of the injury since by this time most sprains should have been much improved. This showed a 'hot' scaphoid indicating that this was indeed a scaphoid fracture and that further splintage (about 4 weeks) would be required.
iv. This case demonstrates the well known phenomenon of the fractured scaphoid with normal X-rays. The fear of missing this injury is common among emergency department physicians although in fact carpal fractures are quite uncommon in children. This is in contrast to the relative frequency of distal radial fractures in this age group. The immature carpal bones are invested with a thick layer of cartilage which is said to protect them and when a scaphoid fracture does occur it is in an older child or adolescent.

Criticism could be made that only the first 3 of the classic 4 scaphoid radiographic views (anteroposterior, lateral, oblique and anteroposterior in ulnar deviation) were taken in the presence of what later seems to be a classic history and examination for a scaphoid fracture. Nevertheless appropriate treatment was given for a 'sprained wrist' and many orthopedic surgeons accept that the thumb does not require inclusion in the cast when treating a scaphoid fracture.

Follow up at 2 weeks is appropriate for such injuries and the decision making process for further treatment is as described above.

The value of repeating the X-rays is two-fold. Firstly the second set will probably be taken in a slightly different plane and if closer to that of the elusive fracture line it will be more likely to show. Secondly, after about 2 weeks cystic changes are sometimes seen around a fracture site. Often, however, as in this case the X-rays remain normal.

Displaced scaphoid fractures which require urgent surgical treatment are usually obvious from the first set of X-rays and are particularly rare in children.

119 An 11-year-old girl presented 4 years ago with sudden onset of swollen wrist joints with no history of injury. This settled but after a symptom free period she developed recurrent joint swelling affecting a variable number of joints.

i. Indicate two important clinical signs shown (**119a, b**), and say what type of arthritis this is likely to be?

ii. What other clinical and hematological signs could she show?

iii. What other arthritides of childhood are there?

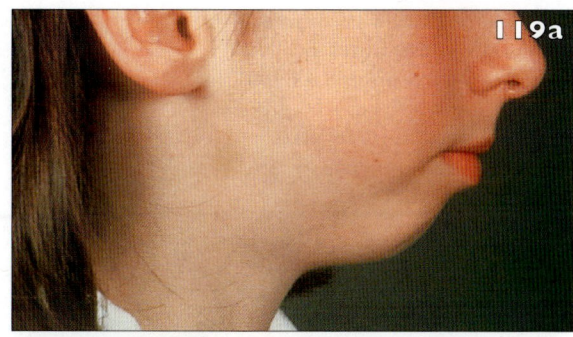

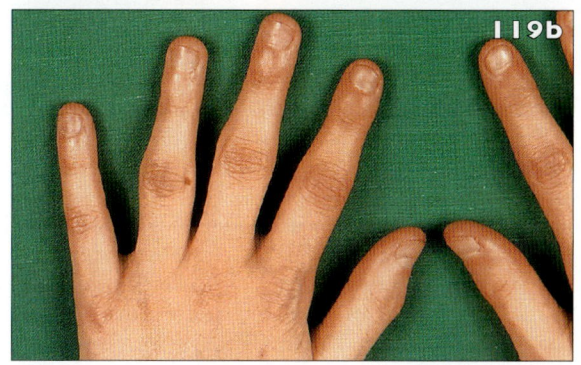

120 A 6-month-old girl presented with a high pyrexia, signs in the left apex, and a raised white cell count. A chest X-ray was obtained (**120**). Describe the abnormalities and suggest a diagnosis.

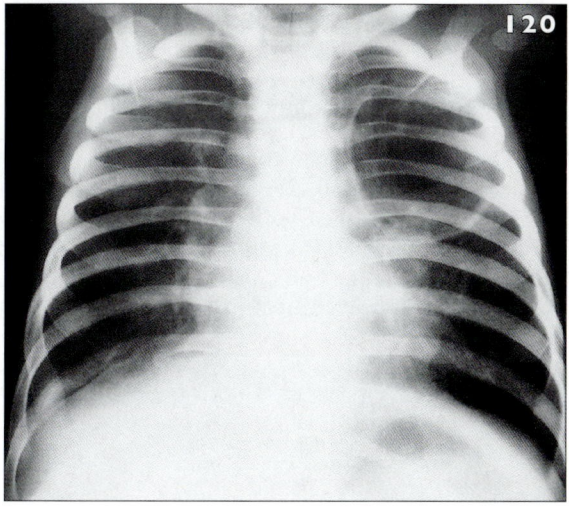

119 i. The slides show mandibular hypoplasia and swelling of the proximal interphalangeal joints. This is likely to be a juvenile chronic arthritis of polyarticular onset and IgM rheumatoid factor negative. Joints commonly affected include the knees, wrists, ankles, and proximal and distal interphalangeal joints. The metacarpophalangeal joints are often spared in this form of arthritis.

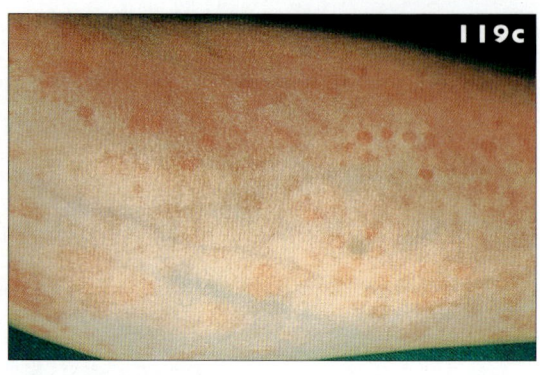

ii. Neck movement and temporomandibular joint mobility are often restricted, resulting in poor growth of the lower jaw and possibly difficulty in neck extension. This may cause difficulty in intubation should general anesthesia be needed.

The blood count often shows a mildly reduced hemoglobin, mild neutrophilia, and moderate thrombocytosis. Whilst rheumatoid factor is always negative, antinuclear antibody is occasionally positive.

iii. Pauciarticular arthritis is present in young girls and iridocyclitis is a feature in about 50% of cases overall and 80–90% of those with positive antinuclear antibodies.

Systemic Still's disease typically affects young children under 4 years of age and produces a spiking fever and a characteristically evanescent rash often coinciding with peaks of temperature (**119c**). This type of disease may be associated with generalized lymphadenopathy and hepatosplenomegaly.

A large joint arthritis associated with sacroiliitis affects boys over the age of 8 years and may be associated with an acute symptomatic form of iridocyclitis. These children often have HLA B27 tissue type.

A rheumatoid factor IgM positive type affects up to 10% of older girls with arthritis. This is symmetrical polyarthritis and affects the metacarpophalangeal joints. Response to treatment is poor.

120 The X-ray shows consolidation in the right lower lobe and in the lingula on the left side, and a thin-walled cavity in the left upper lobe. This is a pneumatocele, which is most commonly seen with staphylococcal pneumonia. The pneumatocele may persist for several months following adequate treatment, but eventually it resolves. Pyopneumothorax can be a complication of staphylococcal pneumonia.

The radiographic features in a patient with pneumonia are seldom helpful in predicting bacteriology.

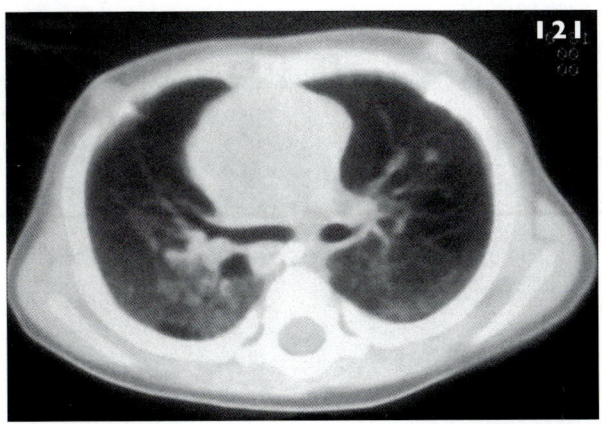

121 A 1-year-old patient was involved in an automobile roll over. She was thrown from the vehicle into a pond. She required brief cardiopulmonary resuscitation at the scene and was referred to a pediatric center.
i. What does the CT scan show (**121**)?
ii. Why is this significant?
iii. What factors are said to affect survival after near drowning?

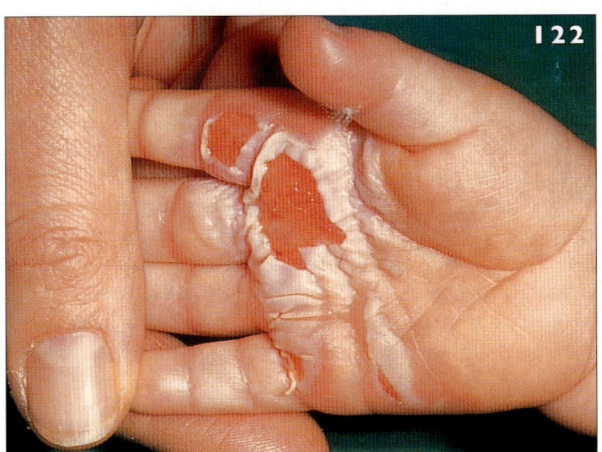

122 This young boy caught hold of his mother's curling tongs and burned the palm of his hand (**122**).
i. Is this history consistent with the injury?
ii. What would be your management of the injury and what complications would you check for?

121 i. The CT scan is of the chest. It demonstrates a small amount of anterior free air, which was not evident on a previous X-ray. The air is central rather than peripheral as is often seen on an X-ray with a significant collection of trapped air.
ii. If this patient were to receive positive pressure ventilation (as she did) the free air from a minor parenchymal injury could expand to a tension pneumothorax and require immediate evacuation. This child, in fact, did develop signs and symptoms of a tension pneumothorax en route to the intensive care unit and required immediate needle thoracotomy.
iii. The outcome in children who have been submerged in water depends on several factors. Orlowski has used five indicators, with one point for each.

- Age under 3 years.
- Estimated maximum submersion time is less than 5 minutes.
- No attempts at resuscitation made for 10 minutes after rescue.
- The patient is in a coma on arrival at the emergency department.
- Arterial blood gas has a pH <7.10.

For a score of <2 there is 90% chance of recovery. For a score of >3 there is 5% recovery.

122 i. The history is consistent with the injury. A young child explores the world with his hands and obviously picks up objects using the palms of his hands rather than the backs of the hands.
Hair curling tongs heat to a high temperature, but are not identified as a hazard by mothers and are often left within reach of young children. A temperature of only 65–70°C (149–158°F) for 1–2 seconds can cause a full thickness burn even in an adult.
ii. The burn has blistered showing a red base, appears to be only of partial thickness, but will be very painful. An antiseptic paraffin dressing applied rapidly will reduce infection, aid healing, and give rapid pain relief by excluding the air. The dressing should be changed initially twice weekly to check for infection and later once weekly. Infection is rare in burns treated within 6 hours of the injury. Healing of an uninfected partial thickness burn in a child of this age should occur within 10–21 days.
It is often difficult to accurately assess the depth of the whole burn in a young child. Small areas of deeper burn may be present in the middle of the superficial areas. These occur particularly at the site of overlying creases of clothing such as elbows where the fabric holds the heat for some time. These are more likely to heal with scarring. If this happens across the skin creases in the hand, it can limit function and may necessitate release later.

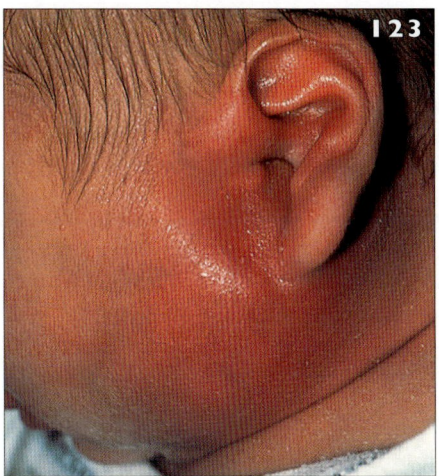

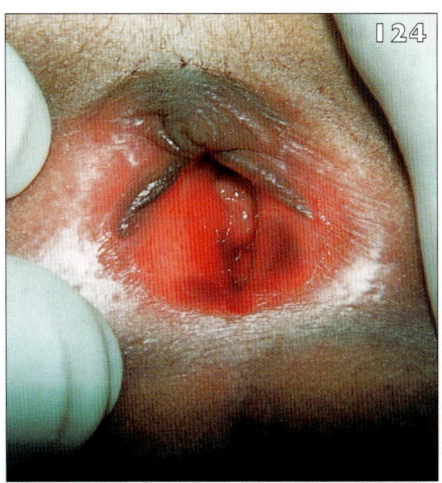

123 This 13-day-old baby developed the appearance shown (**123**). What is your diagnosis and how would you manage this case? What are the hazards of treatment?

124 A 2-year-old presents to the emergency department with a complaint of blood in her diaper (nappy).
i. What vulval findings do you see (**124**)?
ii. How would you interpret the findings?

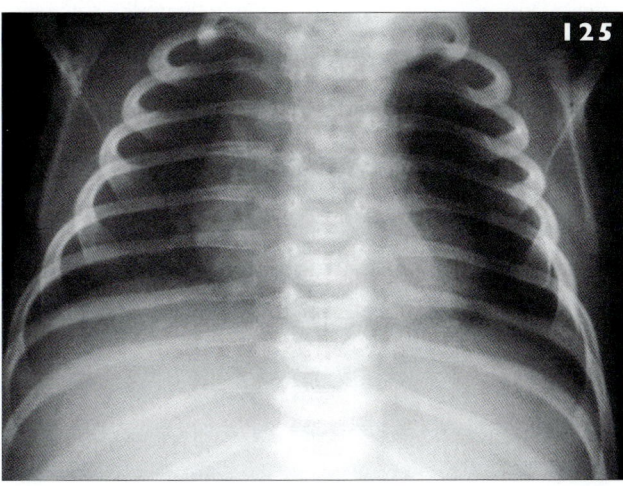

125 A 3-year-old girl presented with tachypnea and fever.
i. What does the chest X-ray show (**125**)?
ii. What is the appropriate management in the emergency department?

123 This baby has acute neonatal parotitis. Pyogenic parotitis is an unusual clinical disorder which is seen mostly in newborn or debilitated older children.

The parotid gland is swollen, tender and possibly reddened. The baby may have a fever and raised white cell count. Expressing Stenson's duct produces a purulent discharge which can be cultured. The most common organism is *Staphylococcus aureus* and antistaphylococcal intravenous antibiotics should be given.

Other treatment is by drainage of the abscess, via Stenson's duct, aspiration through an 18 gauge needle or by incision, taking care to miss the facial nerve which is very superficial in babies. This baby made a full recovery from this unusual condition.

Parotid swelling can occur throughout childhood. The commonest cause is mumps but other causes include a suppurative parotitis, a calculus in the parotid duct, and infections with influenza and other viruses. Chronic parotid enlargement may occur with HIV infection.

124 i. Acute bruising to the vulval vestibule is seen at the 4–7 o'clock positions. The child also had anal bruising, but had no other areas of injury. The likelihood of abuse (either sexual or physical) was great.

ii. Blunt trauma as in attempted vaginal intercourse gives erythema, edema, and even bruising, often lateral to the hymen and also to the hymen itself. The bruising is unlikely to have been caused accidentally. Accidental injuries usually have a clear history and more usually cause bruising or grazes to the anterior vulva, the labia majora or labia minora. Accidental injuries to the vestibule and hymen only usually occur when a child falls on a sharp or protruding object. For children with continued vaginal bleeding, an internal vaginal examination under anesthesia may be required to identify and repair intravaginal injury.

Forensic evidence collection may be helpful in identifying sexual abuse, although little data exists on the usefulness of rape kits in young children.

125 i. There is a denser area behind the heart shadow, with a sharp lateral border. The medial portion of the left diaphragm is obscured.

These findings point to consolidation of the left lower lobe. This abnormality is easy to miss. Always check the diaphragmatic and cardiac shadows for sharpness.

ii. In the emergency department it is important to monitor the oxygen saturation. Oxygen by mask is needed if the saturation is low. In a young child such as this, the most likely causal organism is *Streptococcus pneumoniae* and intravenous penicillin in hospital is therefore the most appropriate treatment.

126 This child's parents noticed that she had facial pain and weakness as well as the finding shown (**126**).

i. What nerve is apparently compromized?

ii. What common childhood malady can be associated with this presentation?

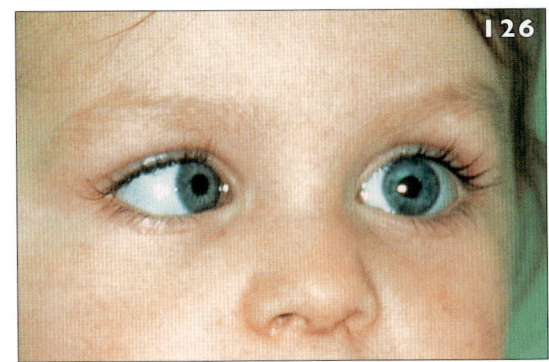

127 A baby presented to the emergency department because of irritability and poor sleeping pattern. The mother had no baby sitter and she brought her other 5-year-old child who had just developed chickenpox.

i. What are the lesions shown (**127**)?

ii. What measures would control his symptoms?

iii. What complications might the baby develop?

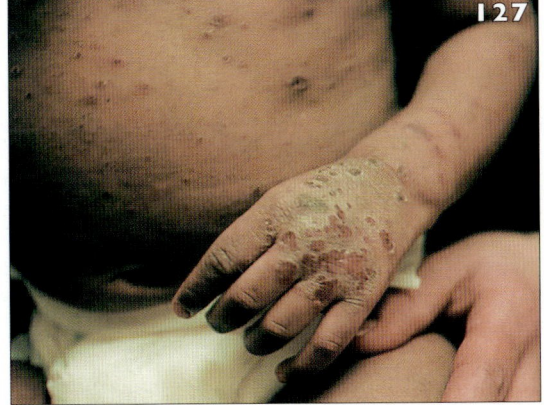

128 This child has bitten through his tongue during a grand mal seizure (**128**).

i. How might this have been prevented?

ii. What immediate problems may result and how should they be managed?

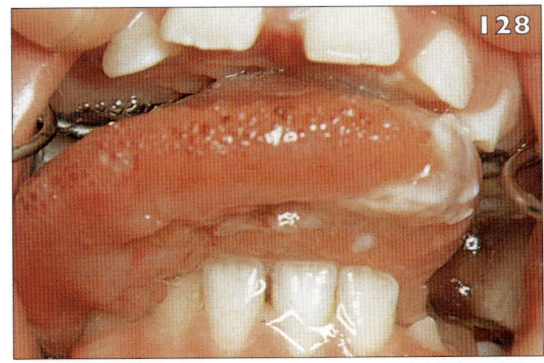

126 i. With the child focusing on an object in front of her face, it is apparent that she cannot abduct her right eye. Failure to abduct the eye is usually a result of a palsy or weakness of the sixth cranial nerve.

ii. In a rare complication of otitis media, called Gradenigo's syndrome, the fifth and sixth cranial nerves are irritated by the extension of the infection to the dura mater overlying the petrous bone. This apical petrositis results in the classic triad of persistent otitis media, diplopia and ipsilateral retro-orbital pain. Treatment of this condition includes intravenous antibiotic therapy and possible surgical drainage.

127 i. The lesions are erythematous, dry, and some are scaly. The rash is suggestive of seborrheic eczema, which usually occurs in infants and adolescents. Many other types of eczema occur in children. The commonest is atopic eczema but other types include primary contact dermatitis, nummular eczema, and dyshidrotic eczema (pompholyx).

ii. This child's symptoms are related to pruritis which causes him to be irritable and to lose sleep. It would be helpful to advise the mother to bathe him in an emollient arachis bath oil, using an emollient soap or similar preparation to help reduce the irritability of the skin. Treatment with topical steroids such as 1% hydrocortisone cream and an emollient would also be beneficial.

iii. There is a risk that this baby may acquire chickenpox from his sibling. Infection of eczematous lesions with varicella virus may lead to severe disease and often the infected eczematous lesion becomes secondarily infected with *Staphylococcus* species. This could result in staphylococcal septicemia and a critically sick infant. This baby's brother was already infectious during the prodromal period of his chickenpox infection; however, it is possible that he had not yet infected this baby. It would be advisable to separate the two children until the older child is no longer a source of infection.

128 i. If the mouth had been propped open with a bite block or an oral airway during the attack the problem would have been prevented. However, a bitten tongue is a rare occurrence in a childhood seizure and it is not generally advisable to place an object in the mouth of a fitting child.

ii. The immediate problems are hemorrhage and edema both of which can compromise the airway. Early consultation with the dental department is necessary as the tongue laceration may need suturing. Nasal intubation may be required if the airway is compromized during treatment or healing.

129 'The treatment of dendritic ulcer (**129**) is topical antiviral agent and steroid eye drops.' Discuss this statement.

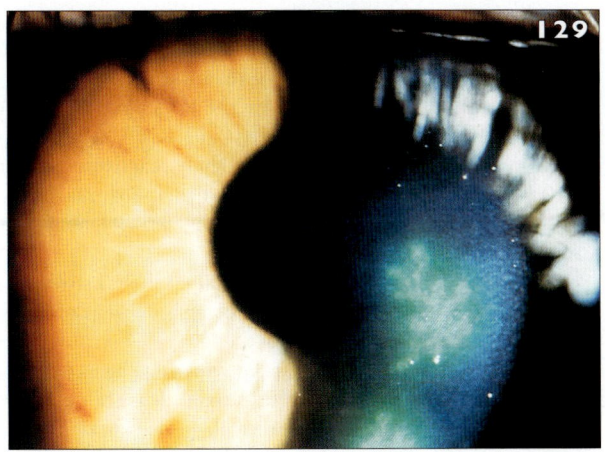

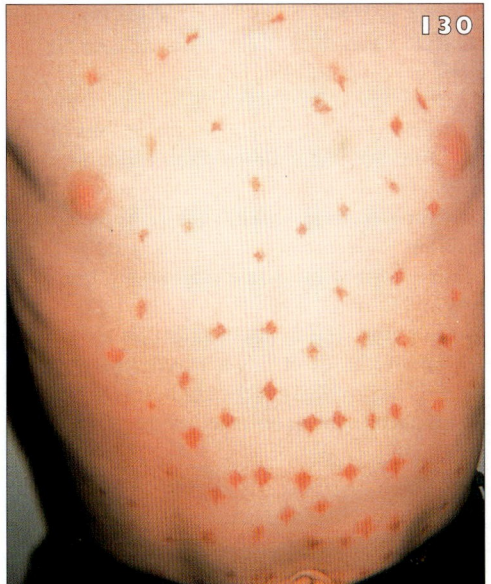
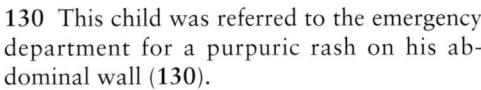

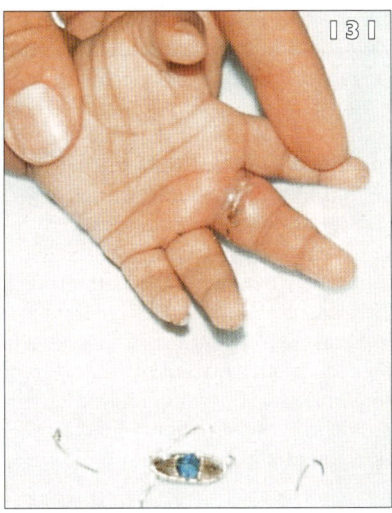

130 This child was referred to the emergency department for a purpuric rash on his abdominal wall (**130**).
i. What is the etiology?
ii. How would you manage the patient?

131 This infant has been crying for the past 2 hours, unable to be consoled by her parents. Examination revealed a painful finger (**131**).
i. What is your diagnosis?
ii. What are your treatment options?

129 A dendritic ulcer is usually caused by type 1 and occasionally by type 2 herpes simplex virus infection. The primary infection usually presents as a cutaneous eruption over the face, especially the mouth and the eyelids, or as a follicular conjunctivitis. Primary dendritic ulcer may follow the follicular conjunctivitis.

After the infective episode, the viral RNA is incorporated within the cell's DNA during the latent period. The virus then reactivates and recurs within the host cells – corneal epithelial cells, or spreads from the dorsal root or trigeminal ganglion cells (possible sites of latent stage) along the sensory neurons – as a result of stimuli from stress, infection or immunosuppression.

The cornea consists of the superficial epithelial surface layer, the middle stromal layer and the inner endothelial layer. The ulcer is an area of loss of the superficial layer of cells. It is branched and has well defined edges. The stromal surface of the cornea at the base of the ulcer is stained by fluoroscein showing the extent of the epithelial defect. The edge of the ulcer formed by the virus infected cells is stained by rose Bengal eyedrops.

Early referral to the ophthalmology department for treatment is essential. This includes debridement by gentle removal of virus infected cells at the edge of the ulcer by a cotton wool applicator and the topical application of an antiviral agent such as acyclovir ointment 3%, 5 times per day for 1 week. Steroid is contraindicated for treatment of dendritic ulcer as the ulceration may become more extensive and geographic or amoeboid in appearance. It is important that all cases of herpetic eye infections should be referred to the eye department for further follow-up and assessment.

130 i. The diamond shape of each purpuric lesion and the pattern of the lesions on the anterior abdominal wall suggest a factitious finding. The child was self inflicting these lesions in order to avoid school.
ii. School phobia can be triggered by a distressing event at school such as bullying or it can be associated with a child who is anxious or depressed and associated with an emotional disorder. The patient and his family would need referral for psychological help and counselling. He is clearly in distress and in need of help.

Signs and symptoms of disease which do not ring true in younger children can be a sign of Münchausen-by-proxy, a condition where the carer has a psychological problem, manifest by manufactured or fictitious clinical problems in the child. It is important to identify the situation and keep the child safe while the carer receives treatment. This is a potentially fatal condition if unrecognized.

131 i. Finger tourniquets can result from many different causes, e.g. rings, hair tourniquets, and key rings. The child was wearing a wire ring that became tightened by movement of a wire band.
ii. This ring was removed by using a ring cutter. The string pull or string wrap techniques are also useful in certain situations. You should determine the technique for removal by the degree of vascular compromise to the finger, any concomitant digit injury, and the material of the ring.

132 A child was brought to the emergency department for a seizure. He was conscious but in a stiff posture (**132**) and had dysconjugate gaze. How would you treat him?

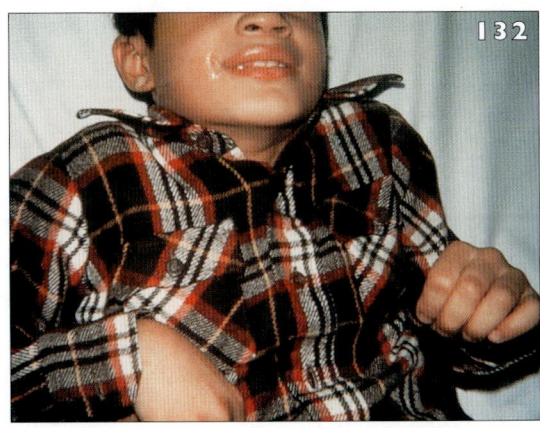

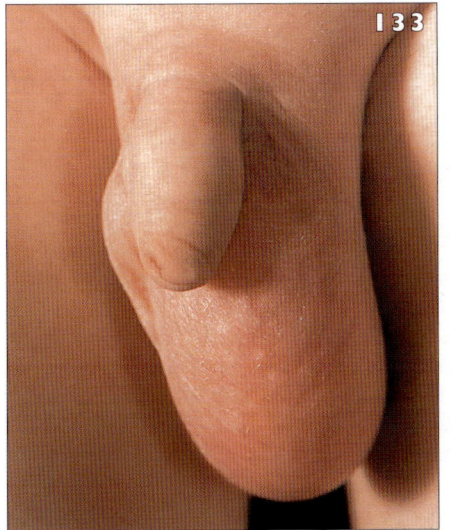

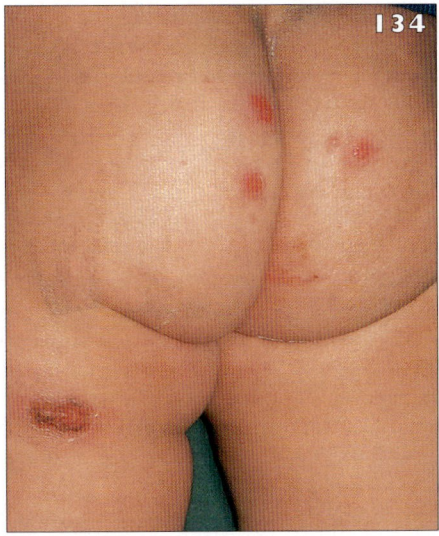

133 This 6-year-old child presented with a painless swelling in the scrotum (**133**).
i. How can you differentiate between a hernia and a hydrocele?
ii. Are there any rare but serious lesions that may look and feel like a hydrocele?
iii. In what way do hernias and hydroceles differ in infancy?

134 This baby presented with a rash over his buttocks discovered after he had been left with a babysitter (**134**). Her mother was worried about the nature of the rash but there was no history of any previous skin problems and no history of injury. What abnormalities do you notice and what is the likely cause?

132 This is a case of some thing that is called a seizure by the parents but in fact is not. It is a dystonic reaction.

Commonly the cause of these reactions is from the phenothiazines and related compounds. There are many other agents that may also cause this idiosyncratic reaction. Moving the child's arm through a range of movement at the elbow will give the sensation of cog wheel rigidity that will support your initial suspicion that this is not a seizure.

The condition should be treated with diphenhydramine 1–2 mg/kg intravenously. This will break the reaction and then oral diphenhydramine should be prescribed for the next few days.

133 i. On clinical examination the area above the hydrocele but not a hernia can be felt. Both, especially in infancy, transilluminate. With a hydrocele it should always be possible to feel the testis, but if it is too tense then it is always possible to transilluminate to see the testis on the posterior wall of the sac.
ii. Clinically, a testicular teratoma can be confused with a hydrocele or hernia. Often the clinical description is 'like a hydrocele but slightly different'. Ninety per cent of testicular teratomas are malignant.
iii. There is no difference between the embryology of a hernia and of a hydrocele. Both result from the processus vaginalis. In infancy a hydrocele is likely to resolve but a hernia will not. In fact, a hernia has about a 50% chance of incarceration if not treated expeditiously.

Sometimes hydroceles are found along the cord in boys – hernia of the cord – or on the round ligament in girls.

134 This child has circular ulcerated lesions of his buttocks and an oval one of his left thigh. They are characteristic of cigarette burns, the round ones of stubbing burns and the oval one of a 'brushing' burn.

Cigarette burns can be caused accidentally or nonaccidentally. Accidental burns are usually single, on exposed surfaces, superficial and often flame-shaped, oval or triangular. Nonaccidental cigarette burns are also usually on exposed surfaces, often multiple, full thickness circular stubbing burns up to 1 cm (0.4 in) in diameter.

Other conditions which can mimic cigarette burns include healed chickenpox lesions and bullous impetigo.

It is always important to listen carefully to the history and assess the whole child. This child also had a circular bruise to her cheek. A child protection investigation revealed that the babysitter had already been convicted of offences against children and on police questioning admitted becoming angry and causing these injuries to the child.

135 This baby who has eczema had a febrile illness and developed a rash (**135a, b**).
i. What is the condition?
ii. How would you treat it?

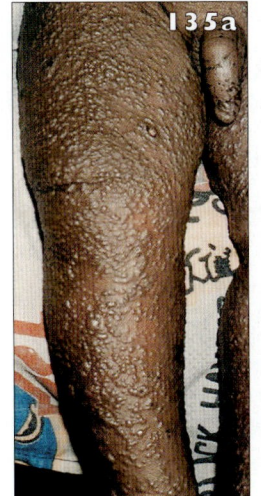 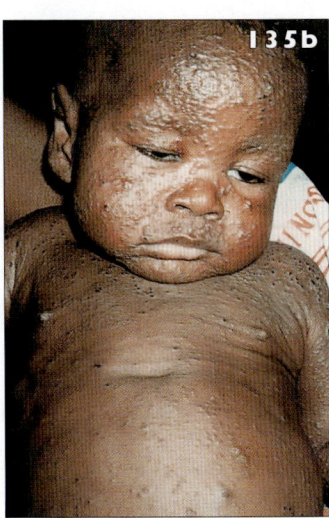

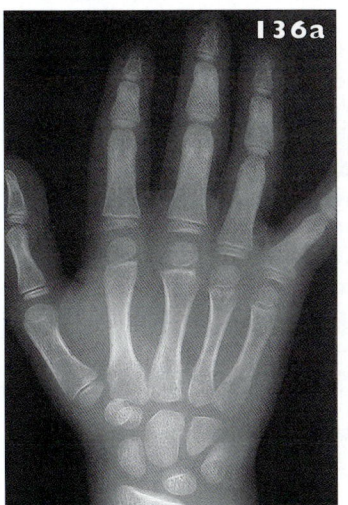 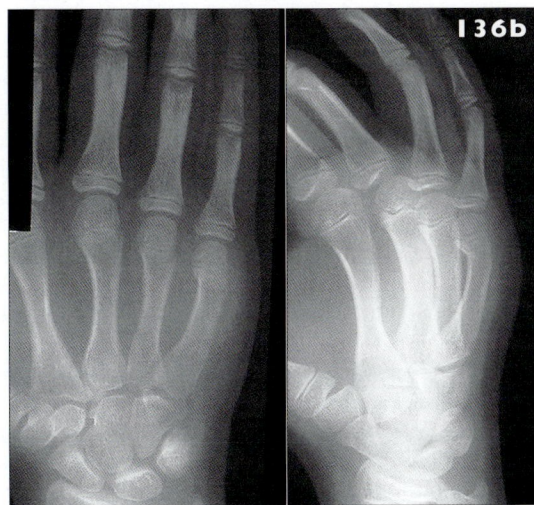

136 What injuries are shown (**136a, b**)? One is much more significant than the other. Describe how you would treat these injuries.

135 i. This baby has Kaposi's varicelliform eruption or eczema herpeticum. This is a superinfection of the eczema by *Herpesvirus hominis*.

ii. *Herpesvirus hominis* can cause a variety of primary infections in children. These include acute gingivostomatitis, acute vulvovaginitis, keratoconjunctivitis, and meningoencephalitis. It can also cause a primary infection of traumatized skin whether a burn, an abrasion or skin traumatized by eczema.

The diagnosis of the herpes virus can be made by obtaining scrapings of the base of a vesicle. The scraping should be smeared onto a slide and stained with Wright's stain (a Tzanck smear). The microscopic finding of epidermal giant cells suggests herpes simplex or herpes zoster.

Children with eczema herpeticum have a constitutional upset followed by a generalized vesicular rash with shallow ulcers most dense in the eczematous areas. There can also be superadded bacterial infection of the vesicles and individual lesions can be mistaken for impetigo or varicella. The child may gradually recover 3–4 weeks after the rash has evolved or further crops of vesicles may occur and the child deteriorate and die.

The eruption should be promptly treated by intravenous acyclovir plus general supportive treatment.

136 In **136a** a fracture of the base of the proximal phalanx of the little finger with obvious ulnar deviation – the so-called 'extra octave' fracture – is shown. The extra octave injury has occurred in the coronal plane. If left unreduced the digit will protrude outwards and impair grip. It is important to assess coronal and rotational malalignment of digital fractures particularly carefully as these significantly influence grip function. The degree of angulation is unacceptable and the fracture requires manipulation. A local anesthetic ring block using local anesthetic without adrenaline provides analgesia. The fracture is reduced by placing a padded ball point pen in the web space and levering the digit back into position over this fulcrum. Another method is to flex the metacarpophalangeal joint to tighten the collateral ligaments and stabilize the proximal fragment while manipulating the distal fragment.

136b shows an example of the so-called 'boxer's fracture', a fracture of the distal fifth metacarpal. It is usually caused by punching someone. The diagnosis is often obvious clinically with pain, swelling, and bruising over the fourth or fifth metacarpal neck and the characteristically depressed knuckle.

This injury, where deformity is in the sagittal plane, requires only symptomatic treatment with neighbor or buddy strapping for 2–3 weeks. Fracture healing is assured and though the depressed knuckle may persist this is of minor significance as it does not interfere with hand function as all the digits continue to flex in the correct way when making a fist.

137 With regard to the injuries shown in **136a, b:**

i. What is the maximum period of immobilization that you would advise in treating hand injuries?

ii. What complications should be considered in **136b?**

138 Describe the fundal findings shown (**138**). What are the most common presenting complaints and diagnoses in a child with this appearance?

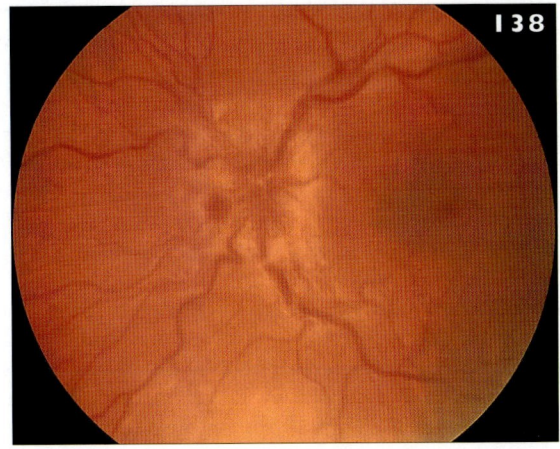

139 A 4-year-old child is brought for care with the problem of a vaginal discharge. Gram stain of the secretions show Gram-negative intracellular diplococci (**139**). What significance does this have?

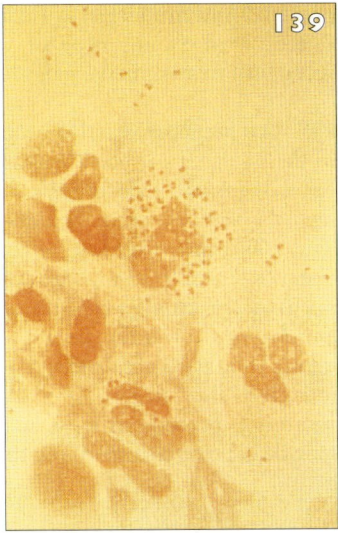

137 i. The treating emergency department physician or orthopedic surgeon should beware of over treating displaced but relatively harmless fractures and prescribing prolonged immobilization (over 3 weeks) which may produce good radiological results but stiff joints. A common aphorism used by hand surgeons is 'to go for function'.

ii. A special case for aggressive treatment of boxer's fractures is where the skin is broken over the knuckles. Careful enquiry should be made as to whether the cut was caused by the victim's teeth as human saliva contains a rich variety of contaminating organisms. If a tooth has penetrated the skin it must be presumed that it has also penetrated the extensor tendon and joint capsule and urgent consultation should be made with the orthopedic surgeon with a view to surgical debridement and antibiotic therapy.

138 This child has optic disc swelling caused by acute papilledema.

Papilledema is defined as bilateral, occasionally asymmetric optic disc edema. Fundal appearances of acute papilledema include congestion and elevation of the optic disc, blurred disc margins, lack of venous pulsations, obstruction of peripapillary retinal vessels, and splinter hemorrhages or soft cotton-wool retinal infarcts on the disc or peripapillary area.

In the chronic stage, it is characterized by progressive visual loss and constriction of the visual field. The optic disc becomes pale, elevated, without a central cup and absent peripapillary hemorrhages and soft cotton-wool infarcts.

Papilledema is caused by raised intracranial pressure, commonly caused by an intracranial mass lesion of the posterior cranial fossa and tumors producing obstructive hydrocephalus. Other causes include benign intracranial hypertension.

The most common symptoms are transient visual obscurations lasting about 5–10 seconds, possibly due to the alteration of optic nerve circulation and CSF pressure, and headaches caused by increased intracranial pressure. The headaches are exacerbated by any type of Valsalva manoeuvre. Transient horizontal diplopia secondary to sixth nerve palsy is common.

139 The prepubertal girl is prone to vulvovaginitis. The level of maternal estrogen falls in the neonatal period. Thereafter through childhood, the hypoestrogenic genital tract has thin atrophic vaginal epithelium and thin attenuated labia minora which do not meet over the vaginal orifice. In addition, fecal contamination can occur from the adjacent anus. Thus most cases of vulvovaginitis in young girls are due to bacterial infections, commonly with *Haemophilus influenzae*, staphylococci, streptococci, and coliforms.

However, this Gram stain is suspicious for, but not diagnostic of, *Neisseria gonnorhoea* infection. Because it is not diagnostic the results of an official culture report should be obtained before taking any further steps. If there is a *N. gonnorhoea* infection, then it is most likely that this girl is a victim of child abuse and child protection procedures must be brought into force. However, other *Neisseriae* species may be causing this stain and the culture will show normal flora.

140 A 4-year-old boy fell on to his head from a 2 m (6 ft) ladder. He was initially dazed and then became awake and alert. Six hours later he presented to the emergency department with vomiting, lethargy, and irritability and was admitted and investigated.

i. What does the CT scan demonstrate (**140**)?

ii. What clinical signs and symptoms would you look for?

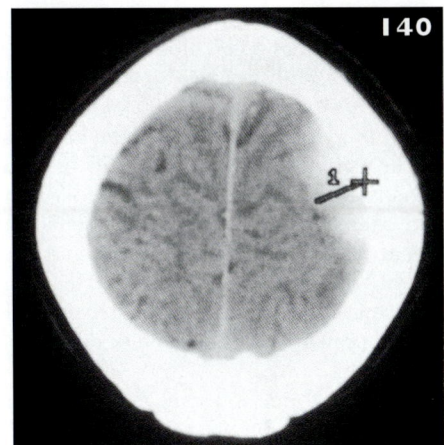

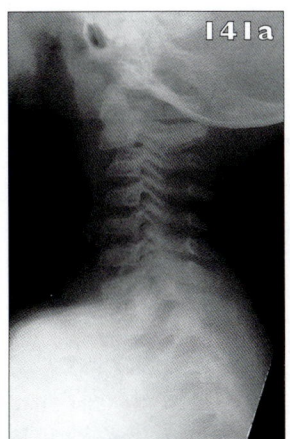

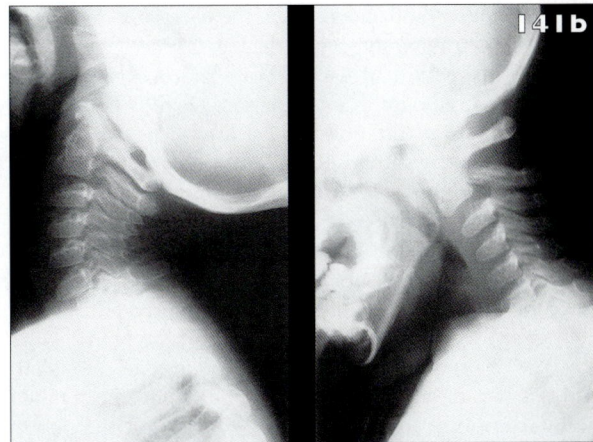

141 Three lateral X-rays of the cervical spine of two different patients are shown (**141a, b**). One of the children has a serious injury; the other does not. What are the respective diagnoses?

The patient shown in **141b** has had flexion and extension X-rays performed. What is the indication for this investigation in the acutely ill patient?

140 i. The noncontrast CT scan demonstrates a typical epidural hematoma. There is a unilateral lenticular blood collection which has stripped the dura from the inner table of the skull, compressing the underlying brain.

ii. This is more often seen in children over 2 years old. It can occur after a major head injury or after a short fall with an apparent minor head injury.

The patient often has a 'lucid interval' after the injury when consciousness, if initially lost, is regained. This is followed by deterioration with headache, vomiting, and altered consciousness, often with contralateral weakness and dysphasia. As the hematoma develops, the intracranial pressure rises causing herniation of the ipsilateral temporal lobe through the tentorial hiatus. Bradycardia, irregular respiration, hypertension, and a fixed dilated ipsilateral pupil develop. A further rise in intracranial pressure gives dilation of the contralateral pupil.

141 Although cervical spine injuries are rare, with only about 2% occurring in children, it is important not to miss potentially lethal injuries.

In **141a** there is subluxation of C2 on C3. There is no evidence of a hematoma in the adjacent soft tissues and no evidence of a C2 fracture. This is a 'physiological' subluxation, or pseudosubluxation, which is a well recognized normal variant. It occurs in up to 10% of children and shows when the neck is X-rayed particularly in those under 7 years old. It is less commonly seen at the C3–C4 level.

Initial inspection of **141b** shows a similar subluxation but when the systematic approach to radiograph examination (see **79**) is used, then on tracing around the axis (C2) a fracture of the pedicle is clearly seen. This is a 'hangman fracture'. In an acute injury the patient should be laid flat and the neck immobilized with a hard collar and sandbags pending urgent orthopedic consultation.

Flexion and extension 'stress' views are performed following treatment of unstable neck injuries to demonstrate return of stability or occasionally under direct orthopedic supervision to demonstrate stability in doubtful cases. It should be emphasized that there is no place for this examination in the acutely injured patient in the emergency department.

In this case the fracture is obvious and the injury is known to be unstable. However, the lack of prevertebral soft tissue swelling indicates that this is probably an old injury and this was in fact the case. Stress views have been taken which demonstrate that there is subluxation at the C2–C3 level. On flexion the posterior spinous processes separate widely indicating associated ligamentous injury and persistent instability.

142 A 15-year-old girl (recent-ly arrived from Africa) had a history of pyrexia and weight loss and signs on examination of the left apex.
i. Describe the abnormalities you can see in the chest X-ray (**142**) and suggest a diagnosis.
ii. What action may you take in the emergency department?

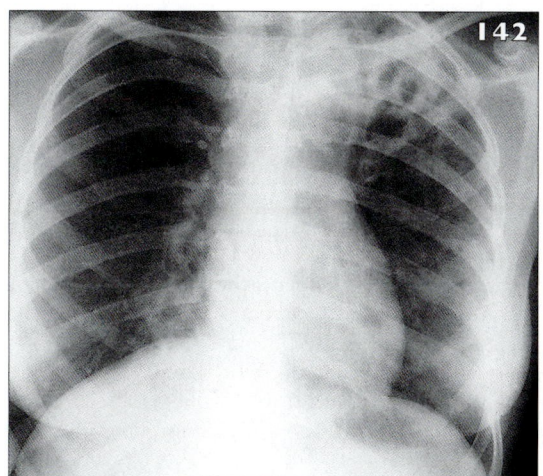

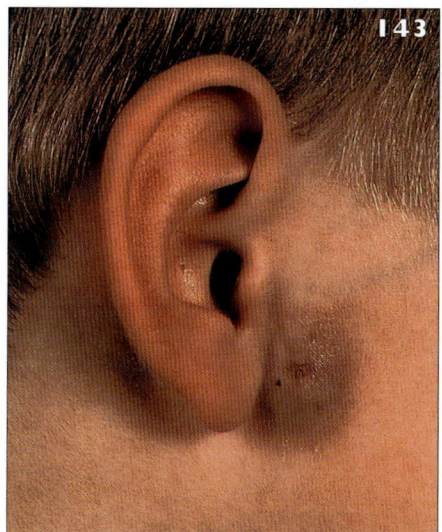

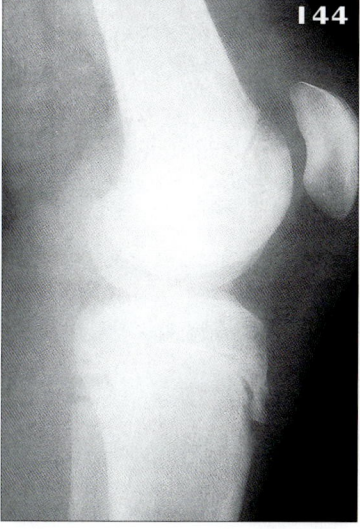

143 This boy has noticed an increasing swelling in front of the right ear with purplish discoloration (**143**). What do you think the swelling may be and what is the usual treatment?

144 A 12-year-old child complains of anterior knee pain for the last 2 weeks. An X-ray was obtained (**144**).
i. What is the likely diagnosis?
ii. Describe the clinical features?
iii. How would you manage the condition?

142 i. The heart has shifted slightly from right to left and the trachea is also deviated to the left. There are thick-walled cavities in the left upper lobe with associated consolidation and elevation of the left hilum. There is left upper lobe collapse, consolidation, and cavitation. These are the appearances of apical (postprimary) tuberculosis.

ii. In view of the cavitation, this child may have open tuberculosis with infected sputum. She should be admitted to an isolation ward and other members of the family should be screened for tuberculosis.

143 The skin involvement, the indolent nature, and the discoloration are typical of a pre-auricular node within the parotid gland infected with nontuberculous myco-bacteria. While resolution may occur spontaneously, the node may break down and form a chronically discharging sinus. Excision of such nodes is curative and there is no need as a rule for antibiotic therapy. The organism is resistant to antituberculous treatment but may respond to a combination of azithromycin and ciprofloxacin.

144 i. This child has Osgood–Schlatter's disease. This is one of the many eponymous 'osteochondritides' in children's orthopedics.

ii. The patient, often an adolescent athlete, presents with unilateral and sometimes bilateral anterior knee pain. Examination shows a swollen tender tibial tubercle. With these clinical features many clinicians feel that radiography in unnecessary.

Findings such as quadriceps wasting and a joint effusion points to an alternative diagnosis.

If obtained the lateral X-ray in Osgood–Schlatter's disease often shows some frag-mentation of the tibial tuberosity (**144**). This is not seen in all cases, however, and this finding is a normal variant in children of this age. Careful scrutiny of the X-ray does, however, show overlying soft tissue swelling which is the hallmark of this condition.

iii. Osgood–Schlatter's disease is generally considered to be an overuse injury and in most cases resolves with rest. In the exceptional resistant case a plaster cylinder can be applied for 3 weeks and the patient should be warned that quadriceps wasting occurs rapidly and takes many weeks to recover.

145 A 6-year-old girl was brought to the hospital by her mother who said that she had fallen downstairs on the previous day. The little girl was withdrawn and would not talk to the doctor. She had bruising of her left forearm (**145**).
i. Why did the consultation raise the doctor's concern?
ii. What examination should he undertake in addition to the examination of the forearm?

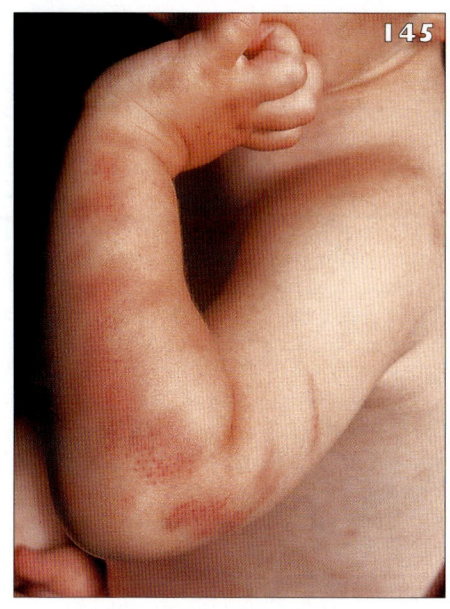

146 A 3-year-old boy was brought in by his pregnant mother because she thought he might have swallowed some of her iron tablets, which he had mistaken for sweets; she was unsure of the number he might have taken. An abdominal X-ray was obtained (**146**). What can be seen in this localized view of the abdomen?

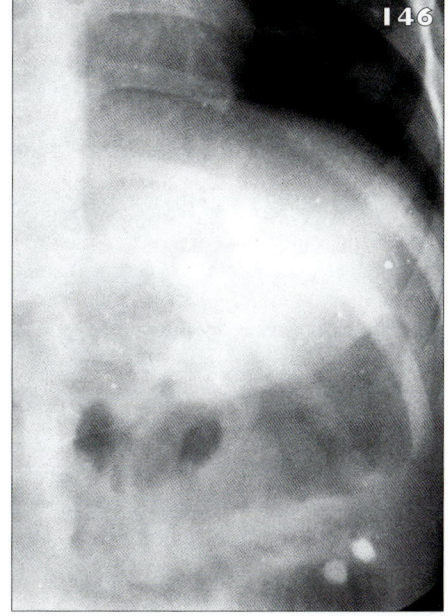

131

145 i. There was extensive bruising of the forearm which did not fit the history of a fall downstairs. The doctor was therefore worried about nonaccidental injury.

ii. A child who is the subject of one type of abuse is at increased risk of other types of nonaccidental injury. The examination of a child with suspected abuse should therefore ideally be carried out by a senior clinician to avoid duplication and should include a social, medical, developmental, and behavioural assessment to try to identify physical, sexual or emotional abuse or neglect. Sometimes this is not possible in the emergency situation, either because of the lack of experience of the doctor or because of the sensitive nature of the consultation. Careful documentation of both the history and examination is essential. It is important to try to work with the parents while ensuring the safety of the child, and it should be only rarely necessary to take legal action to ensure that a child is in a place of safety while a full investigation is carried out by doctors, social workers, and police.

The general physical examination should include height and weight centiles looking for signs of failure to thrive, and the child should be examined from top to toe so that the whole of the skin surface is visualized and the body palpated for tenderness and swelling. This includes palpation of the scalp as tenderness and swelling from a subgaleal hematoma between the scalp and the calvarium can be a sign of severe hair pulling or a fractured skull. This can often only be palpated and not seen in older children who have plenty of hair.

Ears, eyes, and mouth must be observed as these are often sites of injury due to nonaccidental causes. Examination of the eyes including the fundi is essential as they may show signs of both recent and old injuries. Ear injuries do occasionally happen accidentally, but usually in isolation and in a manner which fits with the injury. Ear bruising associated with other facial bruising and ear injuries in babies under 1 year of age may be indicative of abuse.

Bruising must be considered carefully. Accidental bruising occurs most commonly in characteristic sites such as the shins. Bruising of sites such as the inner arms, characteristic patterns such as finger marks or bite marks and bruises of various ages should raise concern. A bleeding and clotting screen should be performed to exclude medical causes for easy bruising. Other marks such as burns and scars must be documented.

Swelling, tenderness or loss of function may indicate a fracture or soft tissue injury. X-rays of specific sites may be required and in the case of a young child or baby, a skeletal survey may be indicated. Above all, if a doctor suspects nonaccidental injury, the child's safety must be ensured while the investigation is carried out.

146 Multiple dense opacities are seen in the stomach and in the left flank. These are iron tablets, which are radiopaque; some are in the stomach and some are in the small bowel. The boy was given the appropriate treatment with desferrioxamine for ingestion of iron tablets and monitored clinically. He was fortunate enough to make a full recovery. Accidental ingestion of iron tablets can be fatal in children if untreated.

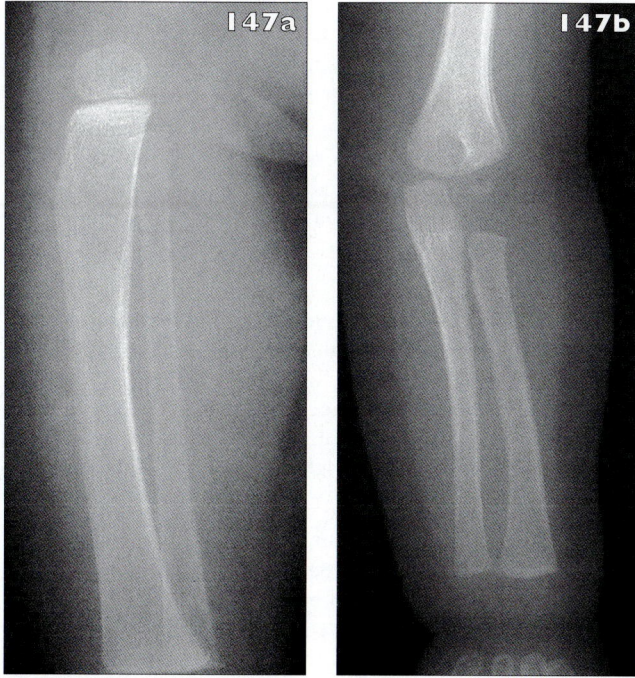

147 i. What do these X-rays show (**147a, b**)? What is its significance?
ii. What should your next action be?

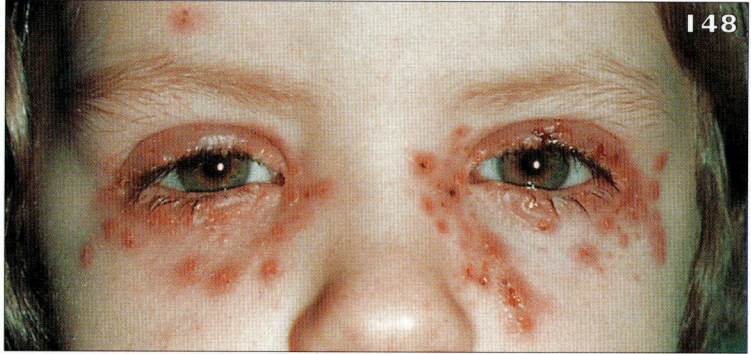

148 What are the likely causes of the lesions on this child's face (**148**)?

If he started complaining of headache, dizziness, and vomiting, what other possibilities need to be considered?

147 i. Careful inspection of the distal tibial metaphysis shows detachment of a rim of bone just above the physis. This subtle injury is a metaphyseal 'corner' fracture and is said to be almost pathognomic of nonaccidental injury. Radiologically it is akin to a Salter–Harris type 2 injury and is caused by twisting with more force than would have been applied accidentally in this 7-month-old child. Diaphyseal fractures are much more obvious and occur much more commonly in nonaccidental injury but when seen they are less specific for this condition.

ii. The diagnosis of nonaccidental injury has far reaching implications and requires a multidisciplinary approach. It is important for the doctor to have clear guidelines and should suspect the diagnosis if:

- There has been unreasonable delay in seeking medical attention.
- The history is not compatible with the observed injuries.
- The history changes.
- There are multiple injuries of different ages.
- There are specific patterns of injury, e.g. spiral long bone fractures in infants, metaphyseal corner fractures, rib fractures, cigarette burns, and retinal hemorrhages.

A detailed account of the history as given by the parents/carers and the visible signs of injury should be documented. A senior pediatrician with knowledge and experience of child protection procedures should then be called.

The child should either be admitted for medical treatment or be in the care of a responsible adult in a place of safety while further medical and child protection investigations are carried out. In this case a radiographic skeletal survey was an appropriate investigation and showed a mature periosteal reaction around the left distal humerus indicating injury some 2 weeks earlier again without any adequate history. A child protection investigation was initiated.

148 Some of these lesions adjacent to the eyes, on the lips and near the nose are vesicular and are suggestive of herpes simplex infection. It is possible that this child may develop herpes simplex viremia leading to meningitis or encephalitis. Neurological examination would exclude any neurological abnormality and the general examination signs of systemic viral infection. Some children require viral studies, including lumbar puncture.

Children with herpetic neurological involvement can deteriorate rapidly with raised intracranial pressure and fits. Some need admission to intensive care units and require supportive management as well as systemic antiviral medication.

149 A 2-year-old girl was rushed to the emergency department by her parents as she was having difficulty breathing and was drooling. She was immediately intubated. The appearance at intubation is shown (**149**).
i. What is the abnormality and cause of what you see?
ii. How is it prevented and what is the treatment?

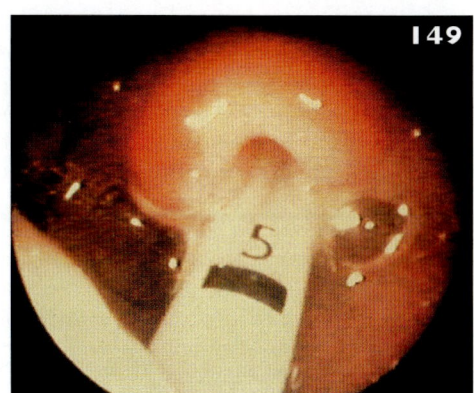

150 This 13-year-old girl presented with a slight and variable facial rash (**150a**), some tenderness in the pulps of her fingers and toes (**150b**), lethargy and recent weight loss. Her hair had become thinner over recent weeks.
i. What is the likely diagnosis?
ii. Describe the involvement of other systems.

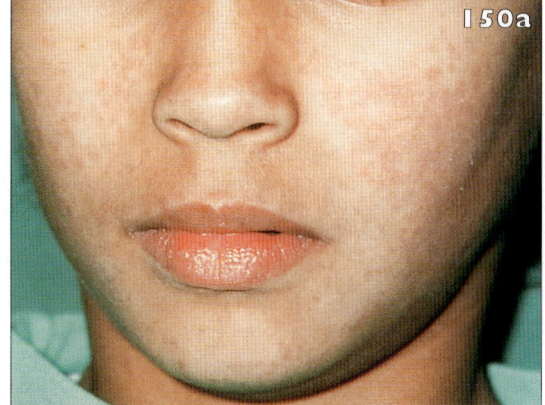

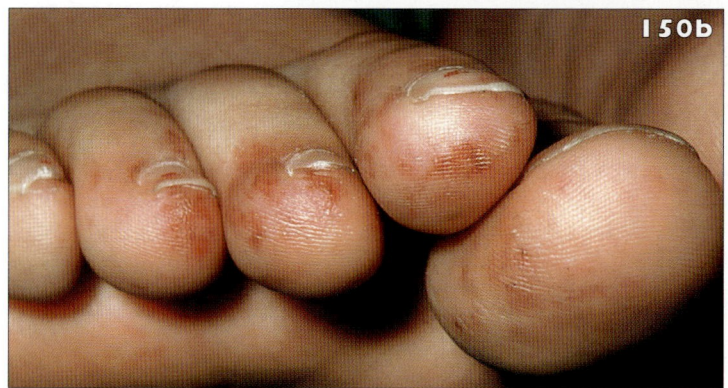

149 i. This child has acute epiglottitis, a rapidly developing septicemic illness involving infection of the supraglottis with severe edema of the epiglottis and pain, usually caused by *Haemophilus influenza* type B. It usually occurs in children of 1–6 years of age. The child looks anxious, unwilling to swallow, dribbles saliva, sits leaning forward to avoid swallowing, and has a 'quacking' type of cough and soft stridor. The child is usually toxic, tachycardic, and pyrexial. The condition may progress with dramatic speed and constitutes a most pressing emergency. Never try to examine the throat of children with these signs and symptoms or undertake any kind of upsetting investigation such as venepuncture or an X-ray of the lateral neck. These may precipitate complete obstruction of the airway, cardiac arrest, and death.

ii. The incidence has reduced markedly since the introduction of *Haemophilus influenzae* type B vaccine but the condition can also be caused by *Pneumococcus* and *Streptococcus* species infection and, rarely, by *Staphylococcus* species. The treatment is by endotracheal intubation by a skilled anesthetist in an intensive care unit or operating room situation preferably with an ENT surgeon present to perform a tracheostomy if necessary. Once the airway has been secured, blood cultures can be performed and the child started on intravenous antibiotics such as cefotaxime or ceftriaxone.

Recovery with the correct treatment is very rapid and the child may be extubated within 24–36 hours and discharged within 3–5 days.

150 i. Systemic lupus erythematosus. This is a multisystem immunologic disorder. The diagnosis is suspected on clinical grounds and confirmed by finding the double stranded DNA antibodies against a wide variety of nuclear, cyptoplasmic, and serum protein antigens.

ii. Renal involvement is common and should be sought as this significantly influences the treatment regime. Joint involvement is common and tends to be relatively mild. Cardiac involvement may be disabling with myocarditis, endocarditis or pericarditis. Pleurisy with effusion may contribute to dyspnea, as may pneumonitis.

Central nervous system involvement may cause fits, confusion or focal vascular lesions. These may result in, e.g. hemiplegia and aphasia.

Skin and joint involvement may respond to treatment with hydroxychloroquine. However, in the systemically ill child steroids are indicated and possible other immunosuppressive therapy. This is usually effective in suppressing symptoms but may lead to serious side effects.

151 A 6-year-old girl presents with a 1 day history of anorexia and lower abdominal pain. She has no fever, has had no vomiting, and had one loose stool today. There is mild tenderness to deep palpation in her lower abdomen.

i. What abnormality do you see on the X-ray (**151**)?

ii. What diagnosis do you suspect?

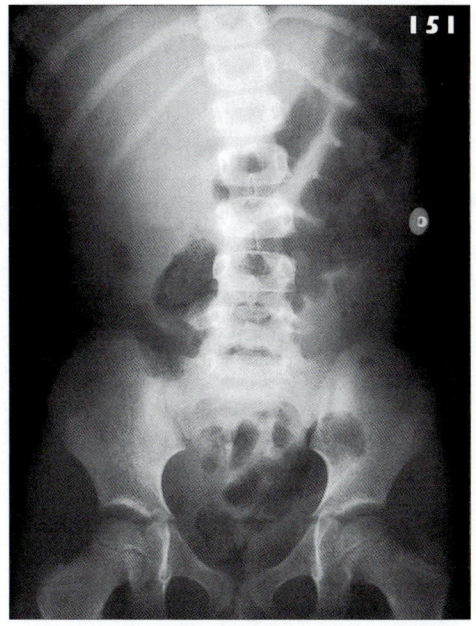

152 i. What possible injury has this boy sustained to his left facial skeleton (**152**)?

ii. What radiographic views are required to reveal the extent of the injury?

iii. What are the options for treatment?

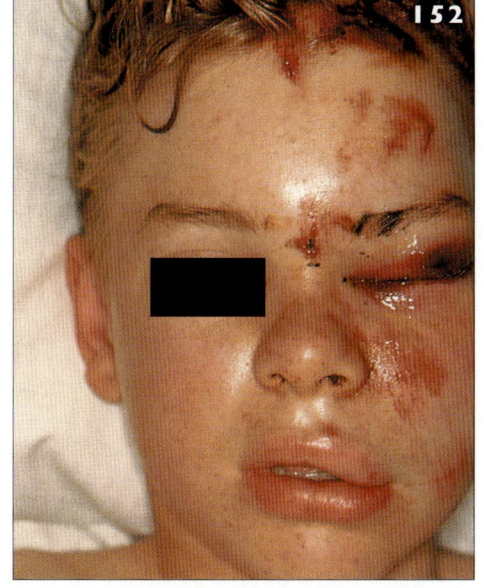

151 i. This is an example of lumbar scoliosis that results secondary to splinting of the rectus abdominus muscles due to pain in the right lower quadrant.

ii. Acute appendicitis is the most common surgical emergency in school aged children. The diagnosis can be elusive, if careful attention is not given to the history, physical examination, and supplemental laboratory studies.

The condition classically starts with mild pain in the right iliac fossa or in the central abdomen, moving to the right iliac fossa. The pain is occasionally colicky, but more usually constant. It is not always associated with vomiting. The symptoms tend to be less characteristic in infants who often present with anorexia, vomiting, and irritability following a respiratory infection. The diagnosis can be delayed and peritonitis is therefore more common in this age group.

The clinical signs are variable. The child may be moderately or severely ill and have normal or raised temperature and respiratory rate. There can be guarding and tenderness, classically at McBurney's point. With a retrocecal or pelvic appendicitis there will be tenderness on the rectal examination. However, this examination can be upsetting for the child and should only be performed once, preferably by the pediatric surgeon.

A full blood count, abdominal X-ray, and urine examination are probably only useful if a urinary tract infection is suspected in the differential diagnosis.

152 i. There is injury to the middle third of the facial skeleton. In this case a malar fracture and LeFort II fracture which separates the central mid face from the cranium. These are usually moderately displaced with some comminution.

ii. The plain radiographic views are 45° occipitomental and lateral facial views. An axial view and CT of the face will also show detailed information of the bony injury and help to plan treatment.

iii. The treatment options are: nonintervention if disruption is minimal or direct reduction and fixation of the fractures using low profile plates. Both options require the child to be reviewed until growth of the facial skeleton ceases. The face continues to grow throughout childhood and growth of the lower face is not complete until the early 20s.

Maxillary fractures are rare in children and are usually associated with neurocranial injuries. They present with malocclusion, facial swelling, and periorbital ecchymoses.

153 This adolescent has restrictive eye movements of the left eye on up gaze (**153a**).
i. What is the most likely site and cause of the problem?
ii. Describe the clinical signs and symptoms in this sort of injury.
iii. How would you investigate and manage the condition in the emergency department?

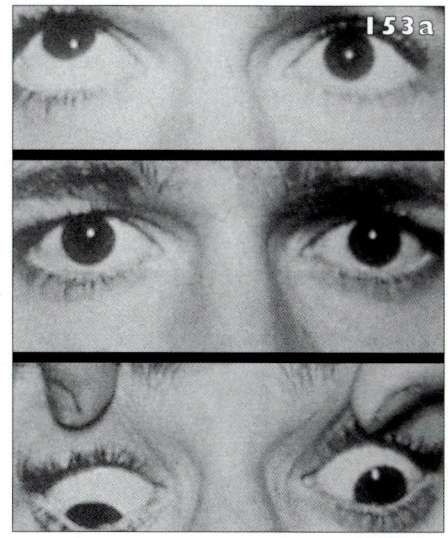

154 A child has been brought to the emergency department with a history of difficulty in swallowing. What does the X-ray show (**154**), and how would you manage this case?

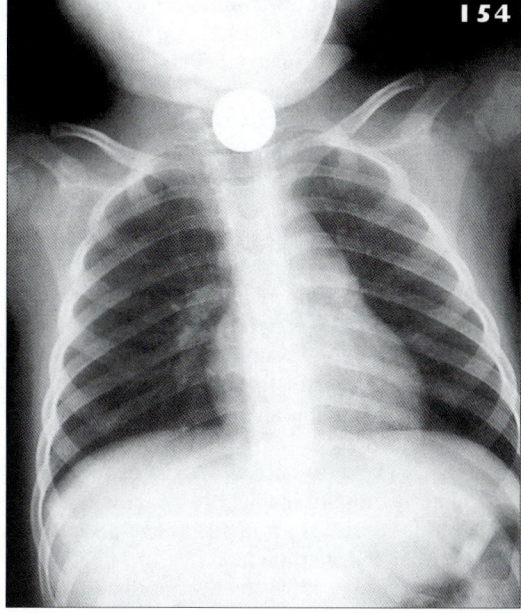

153 i. The most likely cause is an orbital fracture. The sites of fractures at this location in descending order of frequency are floor, medial wall, lateral wall, and roof. The classical 'blow out' fracture is usually caused by a rounded object hitting the globe or the inferior orbital rim. It results from the transmission of force from the orbital rim causing a compression fracture extending into the orbital floor and, or, indirect force transmitted via the globe causing a sudden rise in intraorbital pressure.

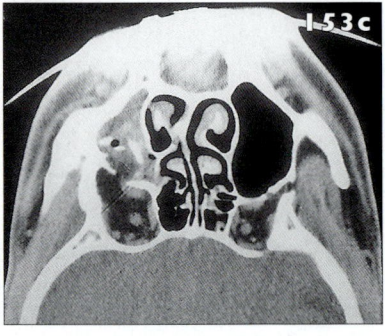

ii. Common ophthalmic symptoms are pain on eye movement, blurred vision, diplopia (usually due to entrapment or paresis of the inferior rectus muscle and, or, adjacent connective tissue in the orbital floor fracture) and infraorbital anesthesia due to injury to the infraorbital nerve.

The signs are periorbital bruising and subcutaneous emphysema with crepitus if air enters the periorbital tissues via a fracture in the maxillary or ethmoid sinuses. Enophthalmos due to herniation of orbital contents through the fracture site may first become apparent when initial periorbital bruising begins to resolve. Retraction of the globe may be seen due to tethering of the involved rectus muscle(s) in the fracture site.

iii. Investigations include a 15° up-tilt occipitomental X-ray to check for fractures of the orbital rim and floor with depressed fragments and the 'hanging-drop' sign caused by orbital tissues herniating into the maxillary sinus. Routine sinus views may show an opacity in the sinuses due to bleeding and occasionally air is identifiable in the periorbital tissues (**153b**). A CT scan of the orbit is the preferred method of radiological assessment (**153c**). Early management should include initial pain relief. Systemic antibiotics may be indicated to prevent orbital cellulitis resulting from infection spreading from the paranasal sinuses. Ophthalmic examination includes assessment of extraocular movements and diplopia, visual acuity assessment, and examination of intraocular contents for evidence of trauma induced complications.

154 The X-ray shows a coin lodged in the hypopharynx. The child is at risk of airway difficulties because of inability to swallow secretions and from progressive edema. Such a coin is easier to remove from its present position than if it passes down into the esophagus where it may lodge at the level of the aortic arch or at the lower sphincter. In a case like this it is usually possible for the anesthetist to remove the coin from behind the larynx following the induction of anesthesia and during the course of laryngoscopy for intubation. It is also advisable to involve the ENT surgeon.

155 A 6-year-old child was examined by a physician after she reported that she had been fondled by her mother's boyfriend.

i. Describe the physical findings seen (**155**).

ii. How does this relate to her complaint of sexual abuse?

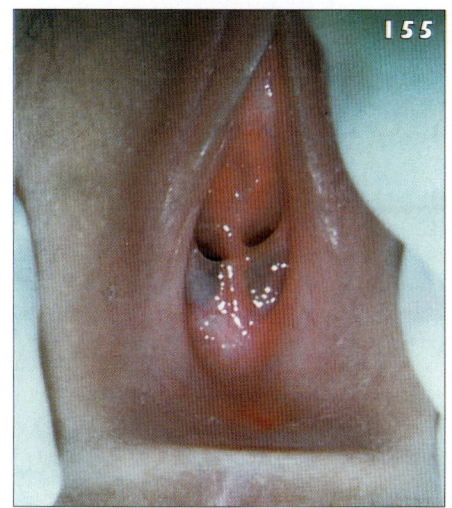

156 This child presented with a rash which started on his face 2 days previously and which progressed downward (**156**). On examination he appeared ill, had a high fever, and a cough.

i. What is the diagnosis and what complications should you look for?

ii. How might this illness have been avoided?

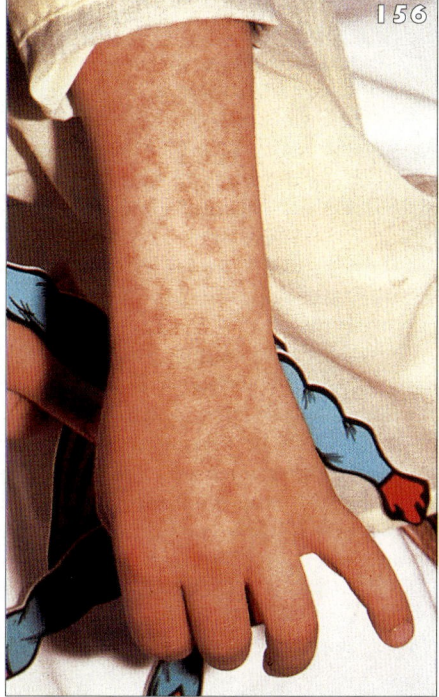

155 i. The examination reveals prepubertal genitalia with a septate hymen.

ii. Septate hymens are an infrequent, but not rare, variation of a normal hymenal configuration. They can result from failure of fusion of the distal Müllerian ducts or incomplete canalization of the sinovaginal bulb, or both. This results in a septum partly or completely dividing the vagina and can extend from the cervix downwards, occasionally associated with duplication anomalies of the cervix and uterus, or the hymen upwards. A septum localized to the hymen is a much more common finding than a septated vagina. If there is a question regarding the extent of the septum, a pelvic ultrasound is recommended. An imperforate hymen is the commonest type of congenital vaginal obstruction and is not usually associated with other congenital abnormalities. It presents as a bulging hymenal membrane between the labia or with hematocolpos.

This finding bears no direct relationship to the child's complaint. However, it is important to remember that a normal genital examination does not eliminate the possibility of child sexual abuse, as this may take the form of touching and fondling, which would not lead to any abnormal physical findings.

156 i. This is the rash of measles in a child who had not been immunized due to his parent's religious beliefs. Measles is a droplet spread disease which is highly infectious from the beginning of the prodromal period to 4 days after the appearance of the rash.

The incubation period of approximately 10 days is followed by a prodromal illness of 2–4 days with fever, malaise, and cough. Koplik's spots develop on the buccal and labial mucosa and disappear in 2–3 days.

The rash develops 3–4 days from the start of the illness and spreads cephalo-caudally. It starts as a blanching red maculopapular rash, then becomes confluent, especially on the face and trunk. It gradually develops a rusty appearance as the capillaries leak and hemosiderin is deposited. It finally fades in 5–6 days. Widespread desquamation may occur about 10 days later.

Complications, reported in 1 in 15 cases include otitis media, pneumonia, convulsions, and acute encephalitis. Subacute sclerosing panencephalitis is a rare but fatal complication.

Measles remains a major cause of childhood deaths in developing countries where malnutrition is common. It is also a danger in children who have immunosuppression, for example during treatment for leukemia.

ii. Measles can be prevented by immunization with a freeze dried preparation containing live attenuated measles virus, usually in combination with mumps and rubella vaccines. This is given irrespective of previous history of these infections. There are occasionally adverse reactions to this vaccine, taking the form of a mild febrile illness about a week after immunization. The child is not infectious during this illness.

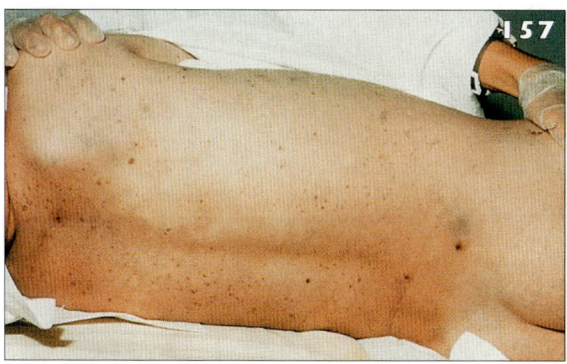

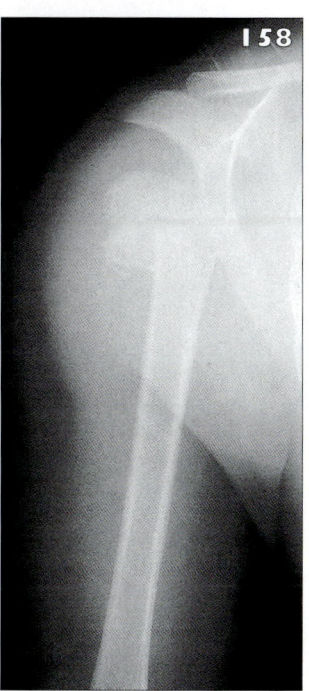

157 This 10-year-old boy presents to the emergency department looking ill with a high fever and a rash (**157**). He is currently undergoing therapy for acute lymphoblastic leukemia.
i. What is the most likely diagnosis?
ii. What is the differential diagnosis?

158 What does this X-ray show (**158**), and how should it be treated?

159 This child has been brought to the emergency department because his mother says he smells terrible (**159**). What is the cause of this?

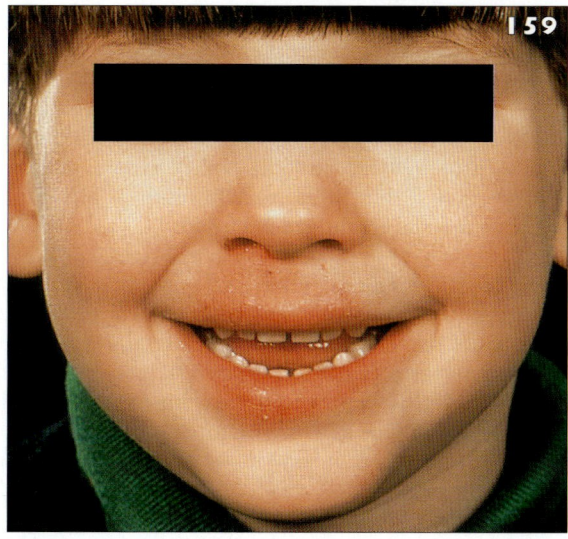

157 i. The most likely diagnosis is hemorrhagic varicella. Classical varicella presents as an itching vesicular rash after a 10–21 day incubation period. The severity of the illness varies widely from an asymptomatic illness to the severe hemorrhagic illness shown. The patient is infective from the febrile prodromal illness until approximately 2 days after the lesions have crusted. The complications of varicellar infections are varied and can affect many systems of the body. They range from secondary staphylococcal infections of the vesicles to hepatitis, arthritis, glomerulonephritis, encephalitis, and cerebellar ataxia.

ii. The differential diagnosis includes meningococemia as well as rickettsial diseases. In the latter, there is an eschar at the site of the mite bites and the lesions tend to be smaller with no crusting. Henoch–Schönlein purpura is unlikely give the extent of the rash as well as the presence of high fever in an ill looking child.

The child should receive treatment for both bacterial and viral infections. Treatment should include a third generation cephalosporin and acyclovir.

158 This is a Salter–Harris type 2 injury of the proximal humerus.

Although the displacement is large, all that is required is a supply of simple analgesics and a broad arm sling to wear beneath the clothing. Children's bones both heal and remodel very well and the younger the better. This 6-year-old girl's fracture will be healed in 4–6 weeks with full functional recovery and the malalignment of the bones remodelled out within the year.

This case demonstrates that fracture reduction is not always needed in children and in this respect proximal humeral fractures are particularly forgiving. Care should be taken, however, when assessing older children and adolescents with such markedly displaced fractures. Fine judgement needs to be exercised in assessing whether the individual is likely to possess sufficient remodelling ability in the remaining growth years to correct the degree of displacement seen. Treatment of displaced fractures by 'masterly inactivity' lies in the domain of those with considerable clinical experience and in this case an orthopedic opinion should be obtained.

It should be emphasized that fractures which enter an adjacent joint and cross the articular cartilage usually produce a 'step' in the smooth articular surface. These injuries heal well but remodel poorly even in the very young and residual displacement of even 2 mm (0.08 in) may result in premature osteoarthrosis. Intra-articular fractures mandate orthopedic referral.

159 He has unilateral discharge with an offensive smell and undoubtedly has a foreign body in the right nostril. The skin of the upper lip is excoriated from the chronic discharge. The offending material is usually either foam rubber from a bath sponge, or vegetable matter. Inert objects such as plastic or metal rarely cause such an offensive nasal discharge and may remain undetected until they form a rhinolith of concreted secretions around the foreign body. Removal of the foreign body cures the offensive odor. A secondary sinusitis may develop.

160 This 11-year-old presented with fever and rash (**160**). He complained that his feet feel ice cold.
i. What diagnosis do you suspect?
ii. What treatments do you initiate?

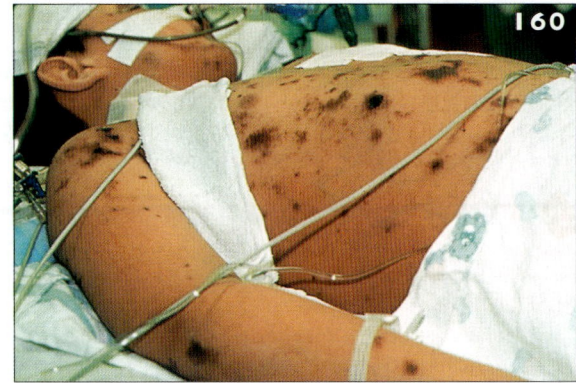

161 A 4-year-old presents for evaluation of prolonged fever for 2 weeks. She has had an upper respiratory tract infection. Her physical examination is nonlocalizing. Chest X-rays are obtained (**161a, b**).
i. Describe the abnormality.
ii. What are the possible diagnoses?

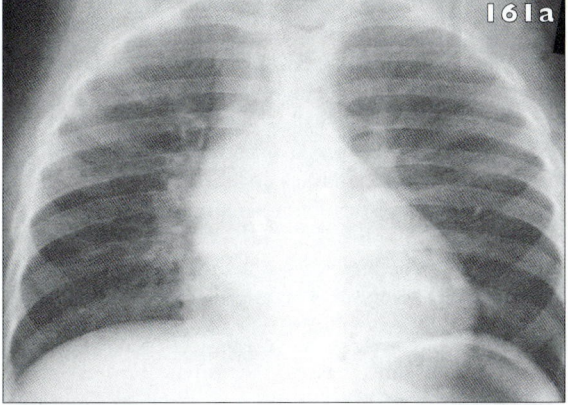

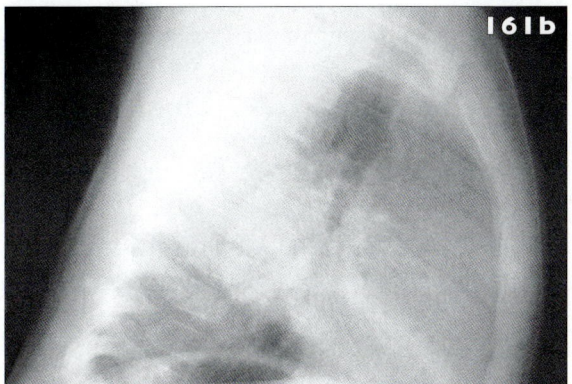

160 i. This child initially had a blanching erythematous rash, but this rapidly changed to a purpuric rash. This patient has purpura fulminans, which is a purpuric rash resulting from disseminated intravascular coagulation and shock with associated tissue infarction. This is caused by endotoxins from the organism *Neisseria meningitidis* and circulating cytokines. Although it can be fatal in less than 12 hours most patients survive. Some of these have areas of skin loss as a result of vasculitis.

ii. A full blood count, throat swab, and blood culture should taken immediately and intravenous antibiotic such as a third generation cephalosporin, e.g. cefotaxime (100 mg/kg) given slowly over 10–15 minutes. A lumbar puncture should not be undertaken in a seriously ill child such as this as it may precipitate coning. The organism may be isolated from the blood or throat. *N. meningitidis* remains sensitive to parenteral penicillin.

Other causes of this rash to be considered include streptococcal infection, measles, varicella, rickettsial disease, and pseudomonal or other Gram-negative rods.

Antibiotics are important, but initially therapies are aimed at the maintenance of vital organ function – the ABC's. Fluid resuscitation in such a patient in the first hours of treatment can have a significant impact on outcome, although too aggressive rehydration can be dangerous. If there is neurologic deterioration mannitol 0.5 g/kg should be given and the child nursed in a head up position.

In cases of proven meningococcal meningitis prophylactic treatment should be undertaken with rifampicin for household contacts.

161 i. The X-rays reveal a posterior mediastinal mass. The mediastinum is the site of most intrathoracic masses in children. The location of the mass is a clue to the diagnosis. The posterior mediastinum is bounded by the pericardium, the posterior ribs, and the diaphragm. The anterior mediastinum lies between the first rib, the sternum, and the inferior surface of the pericardium, and the anterior surface of the upper dorsal vertebrae. The middle mediastinum lies between these.

ii. Common lesions in each area include:

- Anterior: thymic masses, teratomas, bronchogenic cysts, and lymphogioma/cystic hygroma.
- Middle: lymphomas, teratomas, pericardial cysts, esophageal lesions, and hernia.
- Posterior: neurogenic tumors, lymphomas, bronchogenic cysts, and rhabdomyosarcoma.

162 This toddler presented with a spreading rash which was worrying his parents (162). He had just returned from holiday abroad where he had been given antibiotics for tonsillitis.

On examination he had a low grade pyrexia and was unhappy and lethargic. There were no other specific physical signs.

Describe the rash. What is its cause and course?

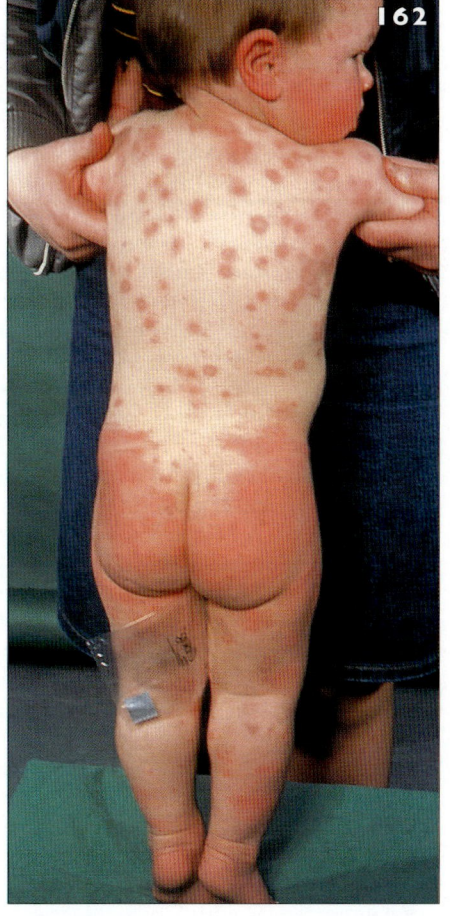

163 A fully immunized 3-year-old child is admitted with stridor. He has had a mild coryzal illness for 24 hours. He has a temperature of 37.6°C (99.7°F). His respiratory rate is 50 breaths/minute with marked tracheal tug and intercostal and subcostal recession. He has a barking cough, and a soft inspiratory stridor. He is agitated and unsettled, and a saturation monitor reads 84% in air.
i. What is the likely diagnosis? What is the likely cause of his agitation?
ii. What is your management?

162 This child has the florid rash of target or iris lesions, predominantly on the limbs and trunk of erythema multiforme, part of a spectrum of diseases from erythema multiforme minor to Stevens–Johnson syndrome. The majority of patients have erythema multiforme minor where the lesions have a red periphery and a bluish center and occasionally become necrotic and bullous. The histology shows a perivascular mononuclear cell infiltrate with some eosinophils in the papillary dermis.

The reaction can be caused by a large range of factors. The most common causes in childhood are drugs, especially penicillins, sulfonamides, and anticonvulsants and infections, especially herpes simplex, *Mycoplasma pneumoniae* and infectious mononucleosis. Rarer causes include immunizations, diphtheria, typhoid, focal sepsis, collagen diseases, leukemia, and radiotherapy.

The rash continues in crops and lasts from 1–3 weeks and may be associated with myalgia. The whole process is usually self limiting but may recur and may occasionally progress to Stevens–Johnson syndrome. Therapy is aimed at providing comfort with analgesics, antipyretics, and antipruritics.

163 i. The combination of markedly increased work of breathing and unimpressive stridor is worrying. It suggests that he has a very marginal airway, with poor airflow. This impression is heightened by his hypoxia, which is almost certainly the cause of his agitation. The underlying diagnosis is likely to be laryngotracheitis, or viral croup. Other causes to be considered are bacterial tracheitis (quite possible with the severe illness), epiglottitis (unlikely in view of full immunization), and a foreign body (unlikely with the history of coryza and the fever).
ii. He requires oxygen, given in a nonthreatening way, preferably given by the parent. He then requires the presence of a skilled anesthetist and an experienced ENT surgeon to assess the need for intubation. Nebulized adrenaline may buy some time while these people are arriving, but will only give transient relief.

Oral dexamethasone or nebulized budesonide have both been shown to be helpful treatments in severe viral croup. Oral dexamethasone has the advantage of being easier to give and cheaper.

Unless there is dramatic improvement with these measures, the child will need intubation to relieve his airway obstruction. Measures such as antibiotics should only be given once the airway is safe, as insertion of an intravenous cannula may upset him enough to precipitate complete airway obstruction. Lateral X-ray of the neck, or examination of the throat are contraindicated for the same reason.

164 A teenager who has asthma complained of a productive cough during the day and at night for 2 weeks. It had disturbed her sleep and she had become irritable and lethargic. An increased dose of her inhaled steroids had not lead to a significant improvement in her symptoms.

i. What signs and symptoms might you elicit on clinical examination?
ii. How would you interpret the findings on her X-ray (**164**)?
iii. How would you manage this child?

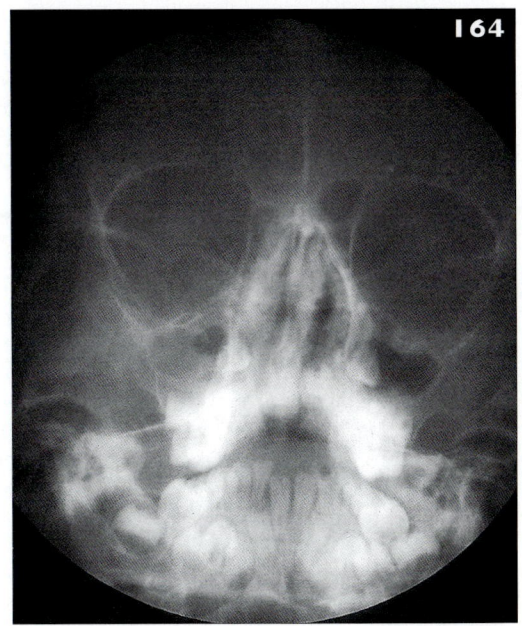

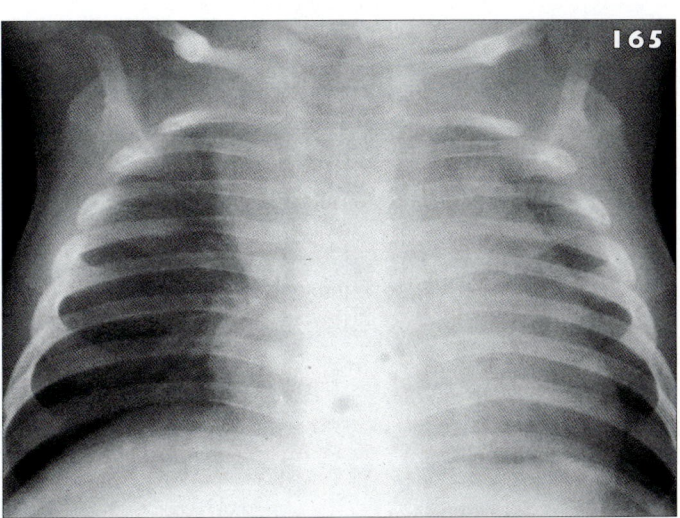

165 A 2-year-old is referred for evaluation of cardiomegaly on a chest X-ray taken as part of a fever evaluation (**165**). What is the diagnosis?

164 i. This patient with atopic asthma most likely has allergic rhinitis. Many of these children develop acute sinusitis (particularly of the paranasal sinuses) with a blocked nose, thick nasal discharge, postnasal drip, bad breath, and headache. They have difficulty sleeping and thus at times develop difficult behaviour. Physical examination may show injected nasal mucosa and percussion tenderness over the maxillary bone. It is important to note that the facial sinuses develop through childhood. The ethmoid is the only paranasal sinus present at birth. The maxillary sinus becomes visible about 6 months of age while the frontal sinus is not visible until 3–9 months of age.

The common organisms causing acute sinusitis are *Streptococcus* species, *Haemophilus influenzae, Moraxella catarrhalis* and *ß-Haemolytic streptococcus* while chronic sinusitis is usually caused by *Staphylococcus* species and anaerobic organisms.

ii. The X-ray shows opacity of the right maxillary sinus. This should be interpreted in the light of the child's symptoms as this can be found in an asymptomatic child with a head cold or with allergic sinusitis.

The maxillary sinus is best visualized on an occipitomental view while ethmoid and frontal sinuses are best seen on an anteroposterior view. The sphenoidal sinuses are best seen on the submentalvertex and lateral views. However, an occipitomental view is usually adequate as an initial request.

iii. This child needs a 2–3 week course of antibiotics such as amoxicillin, or erythromycin if there is an allergy to penicillin. Complications such as cellulitis of the cheek and osteomyelitis of the maxilla occasionally occur.

Topical and systemic decongestants are not very effective. A child with allergic rhinitis would benefit from a nasal spray of corticosteroid preparation or of sodium cromoglycate. The child's asthma control should also be assessed.

165 This is an example of a normal thymus. This organ overlies the heart like an umbrella and is responsible for the wide shadow in the mediastinum. Scalloped or wavy borders are often seen as its shadow joins that of the cardiac silhouette. Typically the rather large thymus in children under 3 years of age produces the 'sail' sign with a wide base narrowing towards the apex, usually on the right side of the heart. Also, in interpreting chest X-rays, remember that the chest radiography is taken as an anterior-posterior film, in variable phases of inspiration and expiration. This accounts for dramatic changes in the shape and size of the cardiac shadow. It is always important to consider the clinical status of the patient when reviewing X-rays.

166 An unconcerned 8-year-old girl complained of a sudden onset of inability to walk. She had no pain.
i. Which signs are important in the assessment of this history?
ii. What are the likely circumstances of this condition if no abnormal objective signs are found and what is the outcome?

167 A 13-month-old boy was presented with a sore bottom. An anal lesion was discovered (**167**).
i. What is the pathogen causing this lesion?
ii. How would you guide further evaluation and treatment?

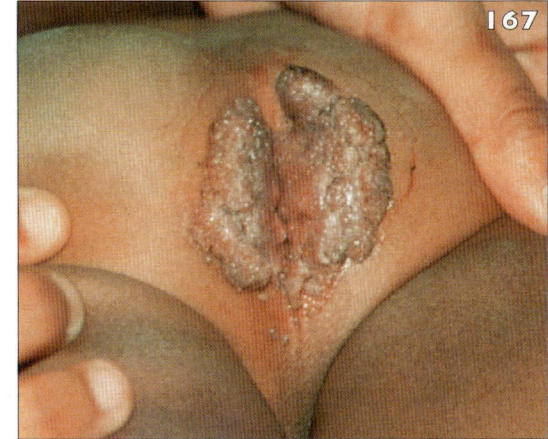

168 An infant was brought to the hospital for high fever, crying, drooling, and some nuchal rigidity. A lumbar puncture was performed and showed no pleocytosis. An X-ray confirms the diagnosis (**168**). What is the critical finding?

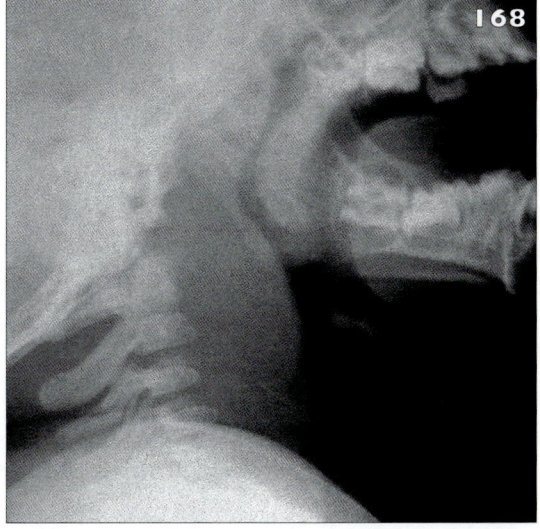

166 i. A full neurological examination is important in the assessment of limb weakness, in particular the assessment of tone, power, and reflexes of both limbs. The child looks indifferent and almost happy, despite her acute inability to walk – otherwise called 'la belle indifference'.

ii. Hysterical limb weakness, or conversion disorder, often occurs suddenly and in response to a precipitating event in the family or the child's wider environment. Assessment fails to demonstrate any objective abnormalities. Often such children also claim that they have no sensation of the limbs when examined. A helpful method of testing for genuine loss of sensation is to ask the child to say 'yes' when they feel touch and 'no' if they do not feel the touch. A child who has no touch sensation cannot say no.

Management often requires admission to hospital for a combination of physical support and psychological intervention. Physical causes for the condition must be excluded. Management includes encouragement to perform activities of daily living, physiotherapy, and referral to a mental health professional. The child usually recovers over several weeks.

167 i. This lesion is condyloma acuminata of the anus. The appearance of multiple flowering pedunculated masses arising from the anal mucosa are caused by human papillomavirus types 6 and 11, which have a predilection for moist skin areas. Large warts in the diaper (nappy) area can cause itching, burning, bleeding, and be susceptible to secondary bacterial infection.

ii. Although congenitally acquired condyloma can be initially noted in children up to the age of 3 years, a detailed history and physical examination should investigate the potential for physical and sexual abuse in this child.

The lesion itself can be removed using podophyllum resin in alcohol which is painted on, and washed off after 4 hours. Treatment is administered every 2–4 weeks until the warts have disappeared. Recurrence after treatment is reported in 20–30% of cases. In some cases, cryotherapy or surgery is necessary. Carbon dioxide laser therapy may be effective when other treatment fails.

168 It is important not to disturb a child who has fever and drooling more than necessary until staff and equipment to support the airway are present. Thus lumbar puncture should be deferred if the airway is compromized in a child such as this and investigations should only be carried out once the airway is secured.

Once the X-ray is taken, it is found to show a retropharyngeal abscess. Note that the prevertebral fat strip is wider than one half to two-thirds the width of a vertebral body. Retropharyngeal abscess may be mistaken for epiglottitis or meningitis, as the children with any of these conditions have fever, are reluctant to move the neck, and they have a toxic appearance. These children usually also have respiratory distress and examination reveals a bulging posterior pharyngeal wall.

The retropharyngeal abscess is now rare and usually occurs as a complication of streptococcal pharyngitis, trauma, or from a staphylococcal vertebral osteomyelitis.

169 This is the chest X-ray of an 8-year-old boy admitted with an asthma attack (**169**). After 12 hours of moderate wheeze he experienced a sudden increase in breathlessness shortly before admission.
i. What abnormalities are shown?
ii. What is the immediate treatment?

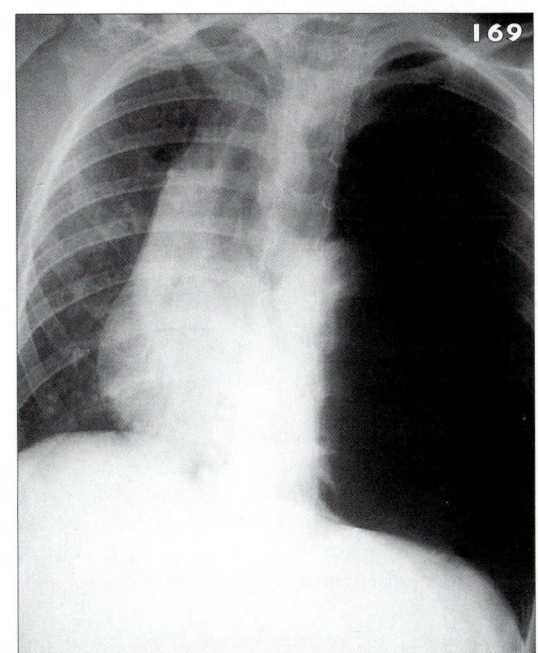

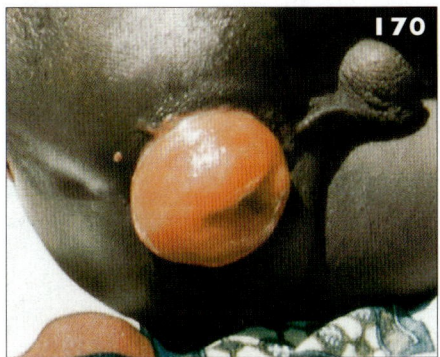
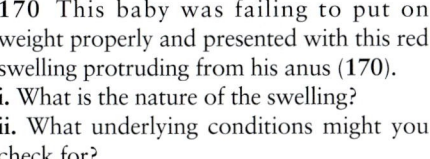

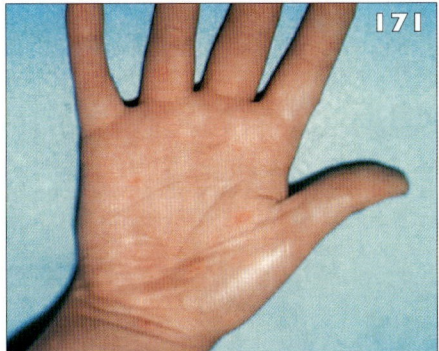

170 This baby was failing to put on weight properly and presented with this red swelling protruding from his anus (**170**).
i. What is the nature of the swelling?
ii. What underlying conditions might you check for?

171 This girl presented with 'spots' on her hands (**171**). She had been slightly unwell and off her food for 2 days with a fever and a sore throat. Which other areas would you examine? What is the diagnosis?

169 i. There is a large left pneumothorax with mediastinal shift to the right.
ii. This is a tension pneumothorax, which is a medical emergency. If there is serious respiratory embarrassment, a large bore cannula can be inserted in the second intercostal space, mid-clavicular line, and left open to air while arrangements are made to insert a definitive intercostal drain with underwater seal drainage.

A pneumothorax is rare in childhood asthma. Other causes include underlying lung cysts, Marfan's syndrome, trauma, and inhaled foreign bodies.

170 i. The tyre or doughnut shaped mass protruding from the baby's anus is a rectal prolapse. The condition usually occurs during defecation and can be reduced after lubrication using gentle finger pressure. Recurrent prolapse can occur and the child's mother can be taught how to reduce it.
ii. Rectal prolapse looks alarming but is not in itself a serious condition. However, it may signal the presence of an underlying bowel condition leading to straining, frequent or bulky stools such as in constipation, diarrhea, giardiasis or cystic fibrosis, or occasionally lower motor neurone lesions such as myelomeningocele. The doctor must therefore undertake a detailed history and examination and organize appropriate investigations to find the underlying cause.

Rectal prolapse is less likely if the underlying cause can be treated and is not usually seen after the age of 6 years.

171 The feet and mouth were also examined. Similar vesicles were found on the sides of the feet and there were lesions on the pharynx.

She has hand, foot, and mouth disease, usually caused by coxsackie A16 viral infection although coxsackie A5, A10, and echovirus 71 have also been isolated from children with the disease. It often occurs in small epidemics and it is very infectious. The peak incidence is in summer or early autumn.

The lesions are characteristically on the palms and sides of the hands, the soles and sides of the feet, and in the interdigital areas. They also occur on the buccal mucosa and posterior pharynx where they may be mistaken for aphthous ulcers, thrush, herpangina, or early herpes stomatitis. The individual lesions are 3–6 mm (0.1–0.2 in) elongated gray vesicles on a red base. They may spread to the arms, legs, trunk, and face and may ulcerate. Systemic illness is generally mild or absent and the eruption clears within 1 week.

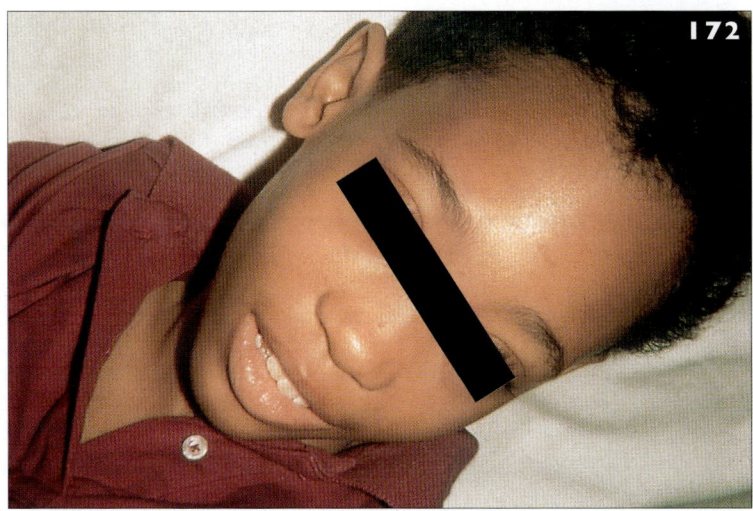

172 This 9-year-old boy with sickle cell anemia is brought to the emergency department with the complaint that mother notices that he is increasingly pale and more fatigued than usual (**172**). What two elements of the physical examination will lead to the correct diagnosis?

173 A child presented with a history of being found floppy and blue in her cot in the early morning by her mother. Her retina is shown (**173**). Is this picture of fundal hemorrhages involving all layers of the retina characteristic of nonaccidental injury?

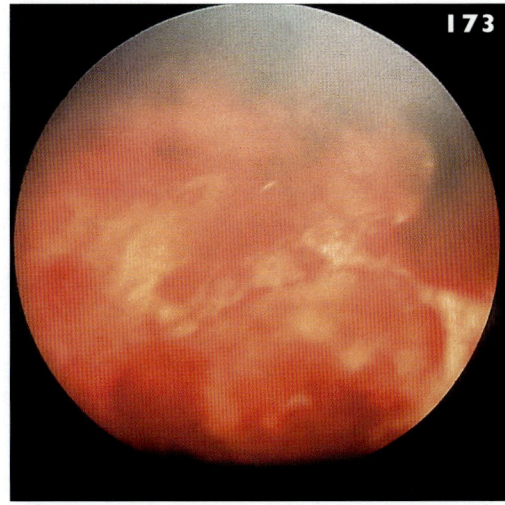

155

172 There may be three possible diagnoses to consider: (1) Hyperhemolytic crisis: these show a fall in the hematocrit, increasing jaundice, and a markedly raised reticulocyte count. (2) Aplastic crisis: these usually follow viral infections which transiently suppress the bone marrow. They may present with fatigue, tachycardia and palpitations, last for 7–10 days and blood tests show worsening anemia and few reticulocytes. (3) Sequestration crisis: these primarily occur in younger children when blood pools in the spleen which enlarges rapidly.

Noting increased scleral icterus points to increased hemolysis. Increased spleen size points to sequestration and the absence of both the findings points to aplastic crisis.

173 Hemorrhages involving all retinal layers are seen in nonaccidental injury. The classification of fundal hemorrhages seen in nonaccidental injury can be divided into the following types: (1) Vitreous hemorrhages appear as curls or linear streaks in the vitreous gel or as diffuse hemorrhage in vitreous fluid. They are seen most commonly in association with severe intracranial injuries. Their onset may be delayed from 1 day to 2 weeks after the initial trauma. (2) Preretinal hemorrhages result from bleeding into the subhyaloid space between the nerve layer and the internal limiting membrane of the retina. They are variable in size near the posterior pole. They appear as a dark red dome-shaped mass and are most dense at the center when fresh. They may gravitate and form a boat-shaped horizontal fluid level. (3) Intraretinal hemorrhages are subdivided into superficial 'flame' retinal hemorrhages from the superficial capillary bed or the superficial peripapillary capillaries, spread along the nerve fiber layer and may resolve quickly, and dot hemorrhages forming small round uniform clusters of red blood cells in the inner nuclear layer, spreading to the outer plexiform layer. (4) Subretinal hemorrhages lie between the photoreceptors and the underlying retinal pigment. They become whitish yellow when they are absorbed. Subretinal hemorrhages come from the choroid and enter between Bruch's membrane and the retinal pigment epithelium. (5) Choroidal hemorrhages occur at the posterior pole and are reabsorbed leaving no trace. (6) White centered hemorrhages are dark rounded hemorrhages with a pale white center.

Examination should ideally take place within 3 days of the injury. Examination using a short acting mydriatic and indirect ophthalmoscopy is preferable especially in an irritable/sick child where it may be more difficult to perform accurately.

Other causes of hemorrhages which must be excluded by examination and investigation include: (1) Neonatal hemorrhages characterized by flame shaped dot and blot hemorrhages, sometimes associated with subconjunctival hemorrhages. (2) Subarachnoid hemorrhages with retinal or preretinal hemorrhages. (3) Leukemia with preretinal, vitreous, and white centered hemorrhages, with hemorrhages in all layers. (4) Blood dyscrasias causing hemorrhages in all retinal layers and in the vitreous. (5) Retinopathy of prematurity with intraretinal and preretinal hemorrhages adjacent to the neovascular ridge.

174 What is the most likely etiology of this child's swollen, painful, cold hand and fingers (**174**)? What is the treatment?

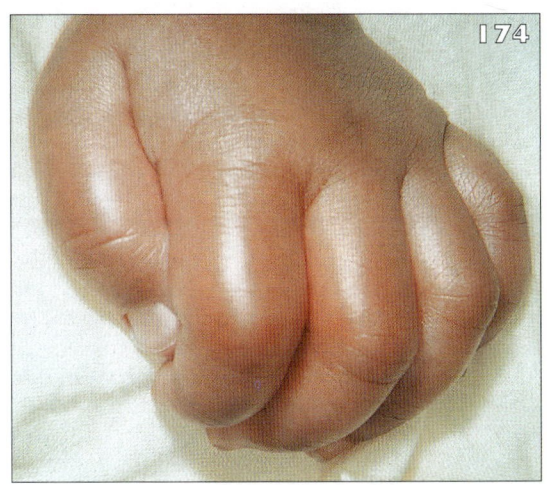

175 An 8-year-old boy was hit by a motor vehicle while on his bicycle. He had no vital signs at the scene of the accident. The child was brought to the emergency department by the prehospital care system. Resuscitation recovered a heartbeat but the patient died in the intensive care unit several hours later.

i. What does the X-ray show (**175**)?
ii. When would you suspect this type of injury?
iii. Would a normal X-ray have excluded spinal cord injury?

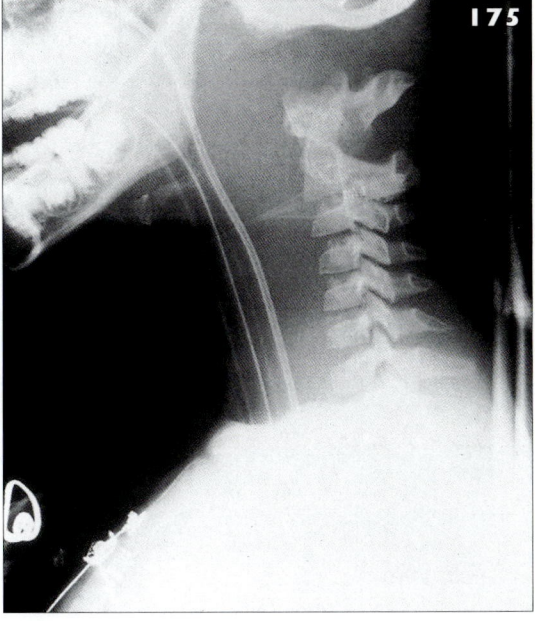

174 This is a hand that experienced cold injury – frostbite. The most appropriate initial treatment is rapid rewarming in a water bath that does not exceed 40°C (104°F).

Swollen red or blue hands and feet (usually to a lesser degree than shown in this picture) are also observed in some neglected, emotionally abused children. It is thought that psychological abuse can lead to severe fear related stress producing hypothalamic deregulation and sympathetic overload. This can result in constriction of cutaneous blood vessels and impaired perfusion. One case has even been reported of gangrene of the toes as a result of emotional deprivation.

175 i. This cervical spine X-ray demonstrates distraction of the occipito-C1 junction. In children injury to the upper two cervical vertebrae is more common. Lower segment injuries are more common in adults.
ii. A high speed incident with rapid acceleration and deceleration may result in a cervical spine distraction injury. The distraction injury seen here is typical of one seen with a high speed injury. One must always suspect cervical spine injury in a patient with multiple trauma even if there is no direct evidence of neck trauma on physical examination. While cases such as this are often fatal, there are reports of survival in children with occipital-C1 distraction injuries.

Clinical features of spinal cord injuries include: neurogenic shock with a combination of bradycardia and hypotension; spinal shock, with loss of cord function after injury with flaccidity and loss of reflexes; abnormal breathing from paralysis of the diaphragm with C3–5 lesions and paralysis of the intercostal muscles with lower cervical and upper thoracic lesions; and reduced or absent pain and sensation masking injury in other areas.
iii. Spinal cord injury occurs less commonly in children than in adults. However, up to two-thirds of children with cervical cord injury have a normal cervical spine X-ray. The greater flexibility of the child's spine, with ligamentous laxity, wedge-shaped vertebrae and shallow facet joints enables it to return to normal alignment after temporary subluxation. Suspicion of the injury alone, whatever the appearance of the cervical spine X-rays, should be enough to lead to management along cervical spine injury protocols with full immobilization and referral to the appropriate specialist.

176 This young girl was noticed to have a lopsided mouth by her mother on the previous day (**176**). What physical signs do you notice? What is the etiology of this condition and what is the long term outlook?

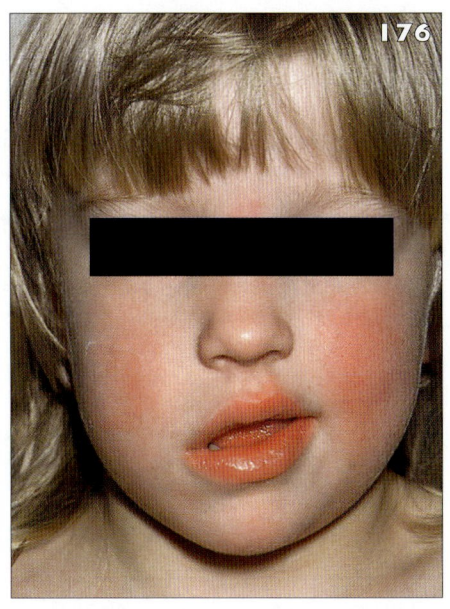

177 A 2-year-old girl is referred for abdominal distension. She was reportedly in a normal state of health until she fell off a bed the previous day.
i. What does the X-ray show (**177**)?
ii. What is the diagnosis?

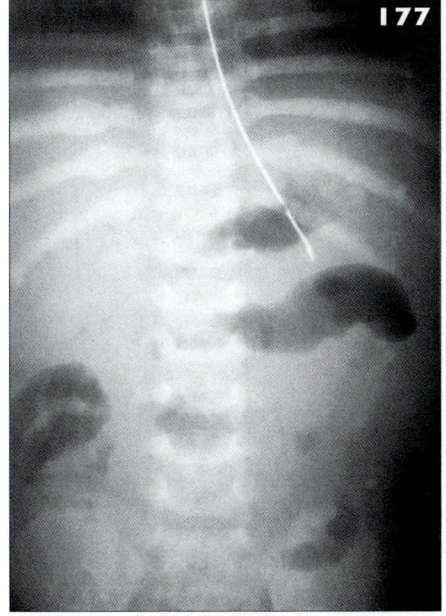

176 She has weakness of the right side of the face – a facial palsy. The usual cause of a facial palsy is a parainfectious mononeuritis associated with many viral infections, especially mumps and which occasionally show tenderness and swelling over the sternomastoid foramen. Lyme disease is the commonest associated infection in the USA. However, there are several potentially more serious causes which must be excluded. Among these are hypertension, middle ear disease, leukemia, and a brain stem tumor. Rarely, it can be a presenting sign of multiple sclerosis.

Two-thirds of cases settle spontaneously, with early resolution starting within 3 weeks. Others are left with only slight facial asymmetry which is only obvious on smiling. Occasionally patients are left with facial asymmetry at rest.

Steroids, if given within the first 48 hours have an immunosuppressant and anti-inflammatory effect. However, they must be given early and in big doses for 3 days tailing off over 1 week. Few children present early and in view of the good prognosis steroids are rarely given.

There is no place for physiotherapy in the management. If the facial palsy leads to incomplete closure of the eye, cellulose eye drops are indicated together with an eye pad during sleep.

177 i. The X-ray shows a paucity of air in the abdomen and old rib fractures, as evidenced by the circular densities on the posterior ribs.

ii. One must suspect nonaccidental injury when the X-ray demonstrates signs of old injuries. In this case the child's carer was implicated in the rib fractures as well as the intra-abdominal injury. This was a ruptured colon, suspected to be the result of an acute blunt force trauma to the child's abdomen.

Abdominal injuries are less recognized as a presentation of abuse than limb fractures, intracranial injuries or rib fractures. They can occur from punches or kicks to the abdomen, squeezing of the abdomen or sudden acceleration or deceleration injuries. There is often no sign of external injury, a denial of any trauma and a delay in presentation. However, a high index of suspicion should be present if there are other injuries or if the child's general condition is poor.

Nonaccidental intra-abdominal injuries reported include perforation of the gastro-intestinal tract, especially the stomach, duodenum, jejunum and ileum, hemorrhage from tearing of major vessels or laceration, contusion of hematomas of liver, spleen, pancreas or kidney.

178 This child has bilateral erythema of her cheeks (**178**). She is afebrile.
i. What historical detail would suggest a benign diagnosis?
ii. What is the pathophysiology of this condition?

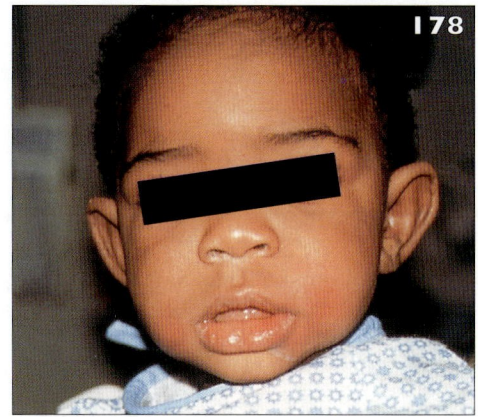

179 This child has fallen and traumatized his premaxilla with apparent loss of the upper central and lateral incisors (**179**). What are the principles of management?

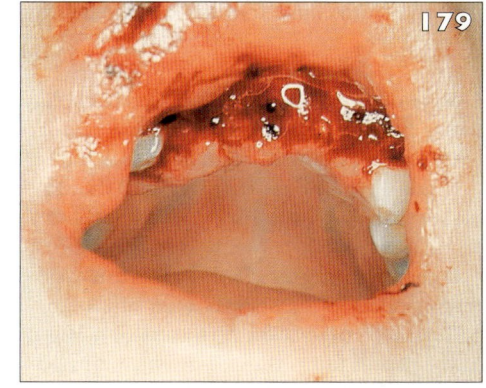

180 A 4-year-old child was playing with her 7-year-old brother, when she slipped while climbing over a dining room armchair. Her parents were in another room when this occurred and did not see the event. When the child went to the bathroom, she noted blood in the toilet and in her underwear. Her genital examination revealed an acute laceration of the labia minora which required suturing (**180**). Her hymen was without injury. Is this injury suspicious for child abuse?

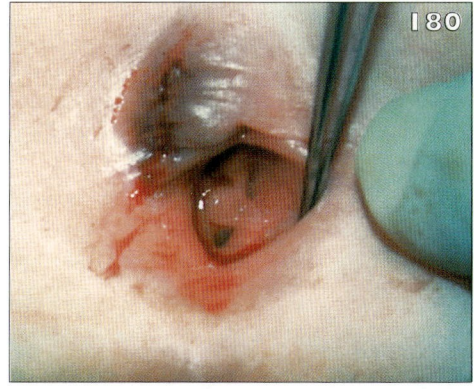

178 i. This child has cold panniculitis. This is a common pediatric diagnosis. In a young afebrile child who appears well but has localized erythema of one or both cheeks, it is important to ascertain any recent contact with a cold object, such as a popsicle (ice lollipop), a cold automobile window or even strong, cold wind.

Fat necrosis of the newborn occurs in the first month of life and leaves several firm circumscribed lesions on the trunk and proximal limbs. The baby remains well and the condition resolves without scarring, sometimes leaving a small dimple at the site of the original lesion.

A more severe condition in the newborn is scleroderma where widespread induration results from multisystem failure resulting in poor cutaneous perfusion. Histology in this group shows edema of fibrous septae without necrosis of fat cells.

ii. Cold panniculitis is caused by the crystallization and rupture of fat cells with subsequent granulomatous inflammation forming crops of reddish purple tender nodules, from under 1 cm (0.5 in) to over 10 cm (4 in) across. In younger children, this tissue has a large concentration of saturated fats, and therefore solidifies at a higher temperature than does adult fat. Cold panniculitis occurs 24–48 hours after the cold injury and resolves over a few weeks. It requires no treatment other than reassurance.

179 Having established that the teeth have been completely avulsed and no bony injury has occurred by clinical and radiographic examination, management depends on whether or not the teeth are available.

If the teeth are lost the wounds should be cleaned and the sockets and lip lacerations repaired by suturing under suitable anesthesia. This child needs a partial denture and as an adult, a permanent prosthesis may be constructed.

If the teeth are available they should be gently cleaned in an isotonic solution and repositioned in the sockets with minimum handling of the tooth roots. They need to be retained in position by means of a splint for approximately 4 weeks. The viability of the dental pulps is questionable and root canal therapy by a dental practitioner will probably be required at a later date.

180 This is a typical straddle injury. It is a common accidental injury in children. When young girls or boys crush the genital tissues between a hard object (e.g. a bicycle bar, a monkey bar, and the arm of a chair) and the pelvic bone, the genital tissue can be crushed or lacerated. Straddle injuries are often anterior genital injuries, and usually heal quickly without the need for repair. The child provided a history that she hit her 'bottom' on the chair and that it hurt.

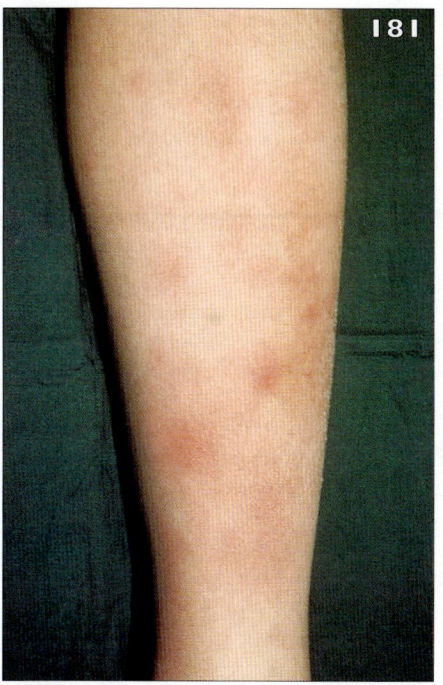

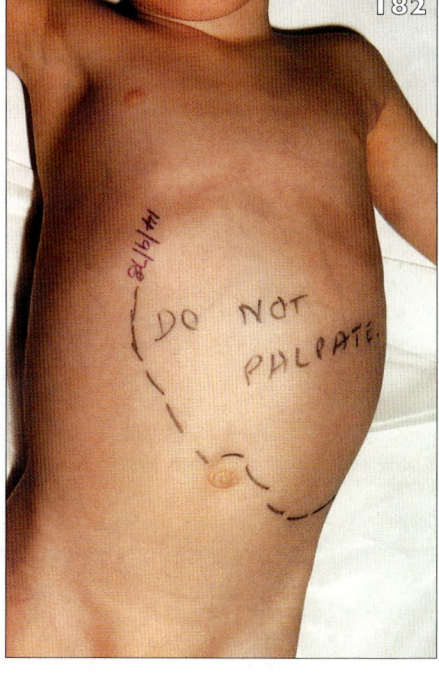

181 This boy presented with 'bruising' to his shins which appeared overnight (**181**). His mother was worried that the doctor would think that she had done it. What is the likely diagnosis? Discuss the possible causes of the condition.

182 The girl shown is 3 years and 2 months of age and had become miserable over the previous 24 hours for no apparent reason (**182**). She would not settle on the evening of presentation and, on lifting, her mother thought the girl's abdomen was tender. The main finding on examination was of a tender left side of the abdomen. The kidney could be quite easily felt.

i. What are the two most likely diagnoses in rank order?

ii. Why should the kidney become so tender with the most likely diagnosis?

iii. In what other ways can this lesion present acutely?

181 This is erythema nodosum, most common in adolescents and rare in young children. It is a condition giving tender erythematous nodules of 1–5 cm usually on the pretibial area but also occasionally on the thighs and forearms and rarely on the trunk and face. The nodules usually last for 1–3 weeks but can occur in crops. If so, the whole reaction lasts for much longer. It is occasionally accompanied by a mild fever and arthralgia.

The histology shows septal panniculitis without fat necrosis, with early neutrophilic inflammation, and later infiltration with lymphocytes, histiocytes and giant cells. Vessels show endothelial swelling and vessel wall inflammation with hemorrhage.

A cause can be found for this condition in approximately 50% of cases. The range of known causes includes infections with streptococci, primary tuberculosis, and *Mycoplasma pneumoniae*, sensitivity to drugs (especially sulfonamides) and foods, and sarcoidosis. Rarely it is due to inflammatory bowel disease, lupus erythematosus, and leprosy.

The treatment of the condition is that of the cause together with rest with the legs elevated and nonsteroidal anti-inflammatory agents. Only rarely is the condition so severe that treatment with oral steroids is required.

182 i. A Wilm's tumor, the most common renal tumor, is the most likely diagnosis, followed by a hydronephrotic kidney. The Wilm's tumor is of embryonic tissue, is bilateral in approximately 10% of cases, and commonly presents from birth to 5 years of age.

ii. A Wilm's tumor may often cause vague discomfort, but acute pain is a fairly common presentation and is likely to result from hemorrhage into the tumor.

iii. A history of recent but often slight trauma can rupture the tumor and cause presentation with acute abdominal pain. Very occasionally, Wilm's tumors present with frank hematuria. However, urinary infection seldom accompanies Wilm's tumors. Infections indicate other causes of renal mass, including hydronephrosis and xanthogranulomatous pyelonephritis.

The treatment of Wilm's tumor sets a model for the treatment of other tumors. The tumor is staged according to factors such as the presence or absence of invasion of the capsule, involvement of regional nodes, metastases, and bilateral tumors. The treatment is tailored to the stage, and thereby its effectiveness is maximized while its side effects are minimized.

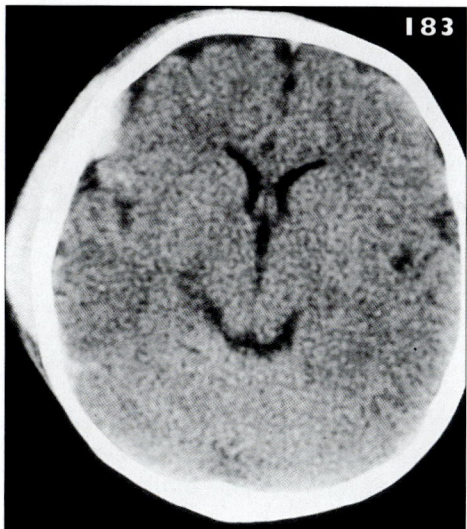

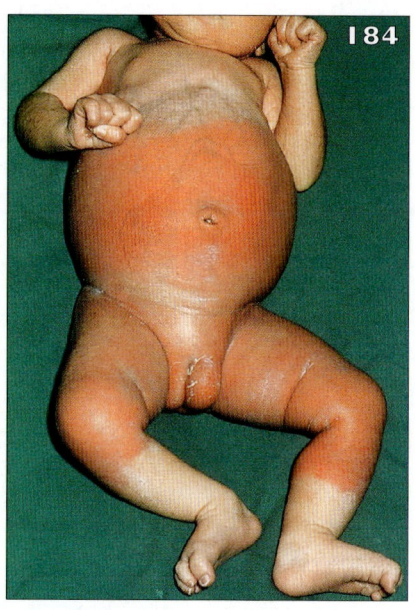

183 A 3-month-old African-American male had a history of having rolled off the bed. Physical examination demonstrated a markedly swollen left side of the face and a very pale child. The child was awake and alert.
i. What does the CT scan show (**183**)?
ii. What is the treatment?

184 This rash developed in an infant who was febrile and irritable for 24 hours (**184**).
i. Describe the rash.
ii. What is its cause?
iii. Suggest a differential diagnosis and management for this illness.

185 A teenager complains of a painful swollen hand after being involved in a fight (**185**). If the child had sustained a break in the skin, what would be the likely cause and what complications might ensue?

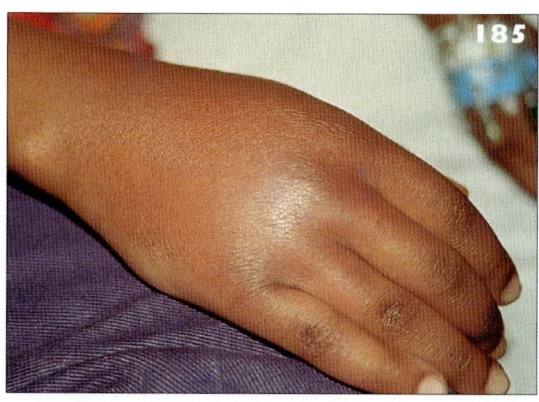

183 i. The CT scan demonstrates an extradural hematoma and an associated subgaleal bleed. The extradural bleed is unusual in a child under 2 years old as the middle meningeal artery, the usual site of the bleeding, has not yet grooved into the overlying bone and is less often damaged by a parietal skull fracture. There is no evidence of intracranial injury or pressure effect as evidenced by normal gray-white interface of brain parenchyma and a symmetrical ventricular system.

ii. As always in traumatized children, close observation and immediate attention to the ABC is the first priority. Special consideration should be given to the circulation to ensure adequate blood volume in a young child with a large blood loss into the subgaleal space.

Thereafter, the intracranial pressure should be lowered using mannitol or frusemide and with the patient anesthetized, paralyzed and ventilated, transfer to an intensive neurosurgical unit should be effected. Hyperventilation further lowers the intracranial pressure.

The definitive treatment is craniotomy and evacuation of the solid clot. In the situation where a general surgeon is faced with a deteriorating patient, burr holes extended to form a craniectomy should be sufficient to save the patient's life, but further surgery will be required later to repair the skull deficit.

184 i. This rash is erythematous and indurated with a sharply defined raised border. Central clearing can occur despite peripheral extension of the rash. The skin is often swollen and very tender. Streaks of lymphangitis can also occur.

ii. The condition is caused by infection with group A ß hemolytic streptococcus. This can be confused with staphylococcal infection and is often distinguished on the basis of skin wound cultures.

iii. Treatment consists of a 10 day course of oral penicillin.

185 This is a characteristic history of an inadvertent human bite when the patient punches another adolescent in the mouth and sustains a small laceration over the third, fourth or fifth metacarpal heads. The hand must be X-rayed to exclude bony injury, (particularly a fracture of the head of the fifth metacarpal, a punch fracture), foreign bodies such as broken tooth fragments, and air in the joints.

The human mouth is heavily colonized by bacteria and over 40 species have been isolated from human mouths and human bites are, therefore, high infection risks. Most bites are colonized by at least five species of mixed aerobic and anaerobic organisms. All wounds must be thoroughly debrided and irrigated but superficial ones may not need prophylactic antibiotics. However, all hand wounds and deeper wounds need prophylaxis to cover both aerobic and anaerobic organisms. Co-amoxiclav or erythromycin together with metronidazole are suitable. A deeper infected wound as shown in this case needs hospitalization, surgical debridement under local or general anesthetic, irrigation, and intravenous antibiotics.

186 A 23-month-old toddler had been refusing to weight bear on his leg for 24 hours. He had been well in himself but had been unhappy and cried when his parents tried to encourage him to walk. He played happily while sitting on the floor or in his high chair. He slept well throughout the previous night. There is no history of fever or of a fall. An initial X-ray was inconclusive. This X-ray was obtained 10 days later (**186**).
i. What is your diagnosis?
ii. What is the mechanism of injury?

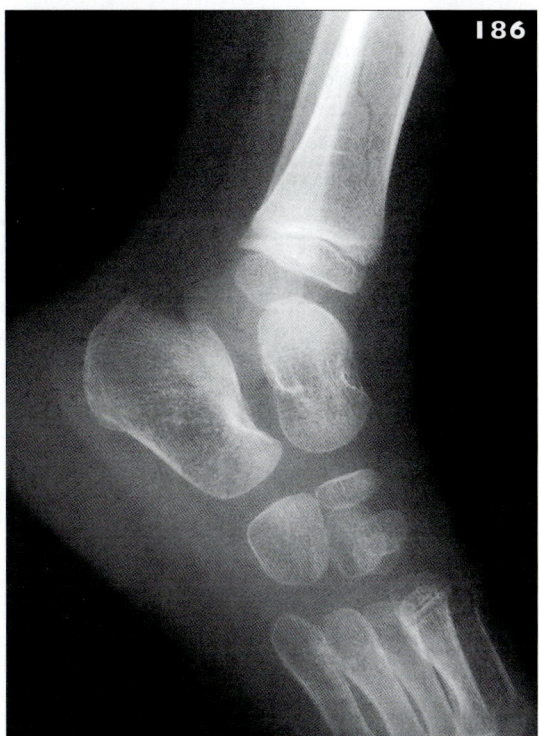

187 An infant is brought to the emergency department in cardiac arrest. External cardiac compression is being performed. Examination reveals the retinal findings shown (**187**). To what do you attribute this finding?

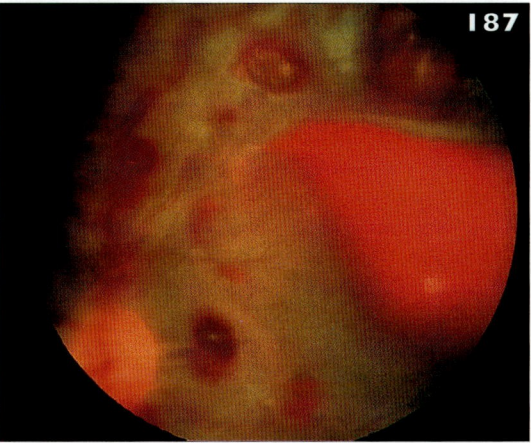

186 i. This is an example of a toddler's fracture. It is a nondisplaced spiral fracture that occurs most commonly in the distal third of the tibia. The history is typical of this type of fracture in an active toddler with no specific episode of falling or other trauma. The physical signs can also be misleading as the only positive clinical signs are a reluctance to weight bear and slightly increased warmth over the lower tibia. Occasionally there may be a slight withdrawal of the limb on direct pressure over the fracture site. There is usually no evidence of bruising or swelling.

X-rays may also be misleading as the fracture may not show on an X-ray taken within a day of the fracture. X-rays 10 days later may reveal either the fracture or some periosteal reaction around the fracture site (**186**).
ii. This type of fracture results from a rotational force applied to the porous pediatric bone. This can happen accidentally in a twisting fall. It can also happen if the leg is grasped firmly and twisted in a nonaccidental injury.

187 The finding of acute retinal hemorrhage is caused by trauma. Retinal hemorrhages are not the result of external cardiac compression in the resuscitation of a collapsed child. They do occur in approximately 10% of newborn babies but these rapidly disappear a few days after birth. If there is no history of trauma, child abuse must be excluded.

In child abuse, retinal hemorrhages can be caused by a direct blow to the head or from a shaking injury associated with chest compression as the child is held gripping the chest wall forcibly. It is thought that the grip can be so forceful that the cranial intravenous pressure is raised, compressing the retinal vein leading to rupture of the intraretinal capillaries which leak into the retina. A tight grip can also cause fractured ribs. The hemorrhages are most frequent in the anterior part of the eye. They are, therefore, difficult to see by direct fundoscopy and examination by an ophthalmologist is required.

Other than in the neonatal period, babies with retinal hemorrhages require admission and thorough investigation including CT scan of the brain, a bleeding and clotting screen, and a skeletal survey.

188 What is the lesion of this boy's knee (**188**)? How would you treat it and what advice would you give the boy's parents on hygiene?

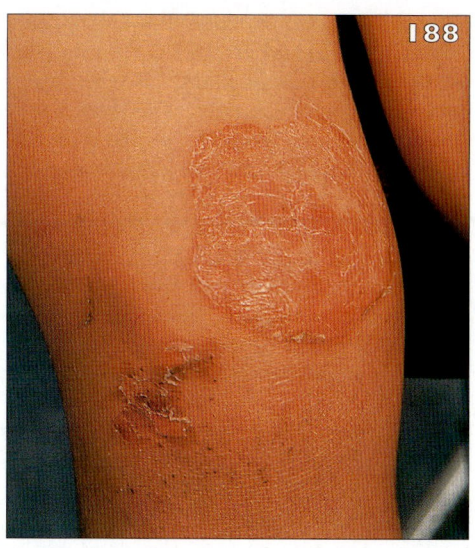

189 An X-ray of the chest and abdomen of a baby presented as a 'collapse' is shown (**189a**). She had a distended abdomen and was resuscitated. What can you see?

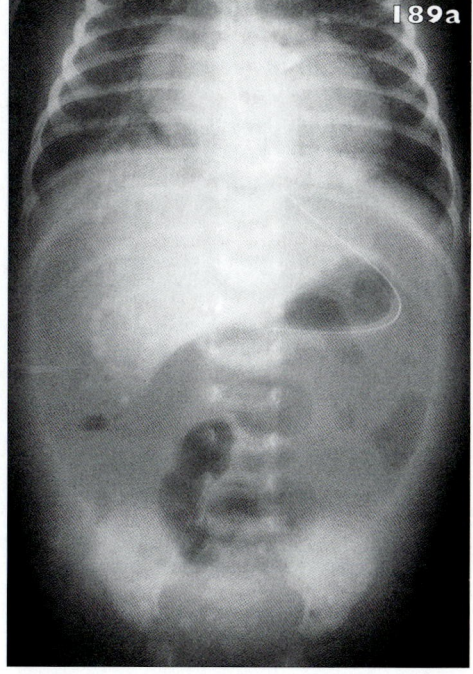

188 This boy has impetigo of his knee. This is a superficial skin infection caused by a *Staphylococcus aureus* and occasionally by a streptococcal infection. The bullae, usually of the face or limbs, fill with pus and then rupture leaving superficial ulcers which ooze and then crust. The lesions may spread both locally and diffusely. Local lymph nodes may become swollen and inflamed. The disease can present in several guises. If flaccid bullae are present the condition is called bullous impetigo and is caused by an epidermolytic toxin producing strain of *S. aureus*.

It is highly infectious and can occasionally occur as a secondary infection in a child with scabies, herpes simplex, dermatitis, or insect bites and abrasions. Cases which are refractory to treatment should be checked for an underlying condition. Bacterial folliculitis can occur on the scalp associated with hair under tension, e.g. braided plaits. It is treated by releasing tension on the hair.

The child should be treated promptly and isolated as far as possible. He should certainly have separate flannels and towels from other people. Cetrimide and saline washes together with antistaphylococcal antibiotic creams are effective in mild cases. Occasionally in severe cases, an oral antibiotic is needed.

189 There are signs of a pneumoperitoneum. The free air is outlined by the small arrowheads in **189b**, giving an 'American football sign'. The falciform ligament, which stretches from the liver to the umbilicus, is also seen. This can only occur when free air is present in the peritoneal cavity (large arrow). The child is lying on its back and the free air rises anteriorly. These are the signs of pneumoperitoneum on a supine film.

In a sick small child, a cross table decubitus film, with the baby lying with its left side down, confirms whether or not there is a pneumoperitoneum. In older children an erect chest film is more useful.

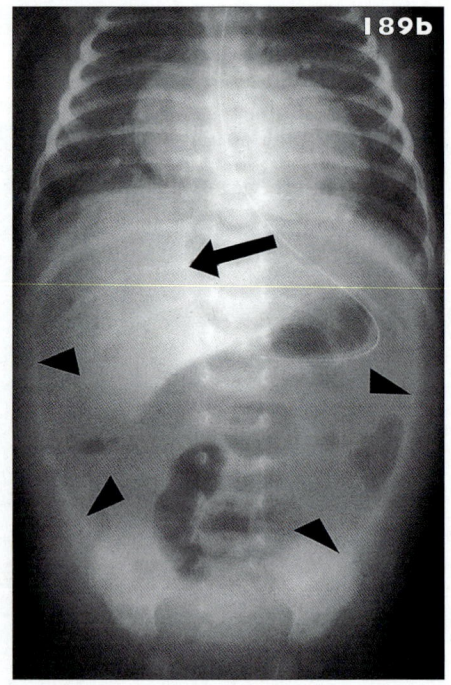

189b

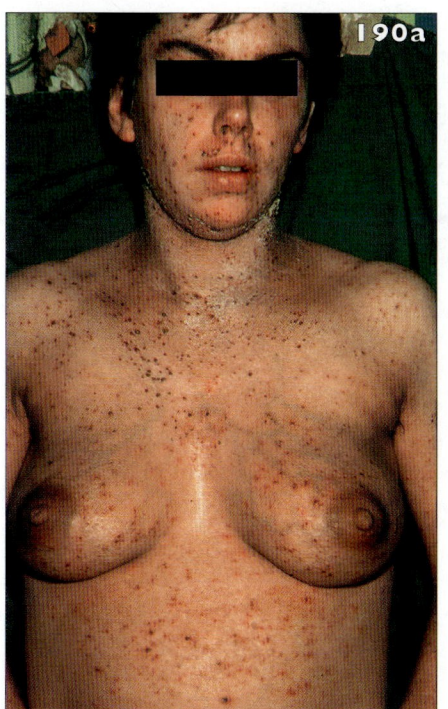

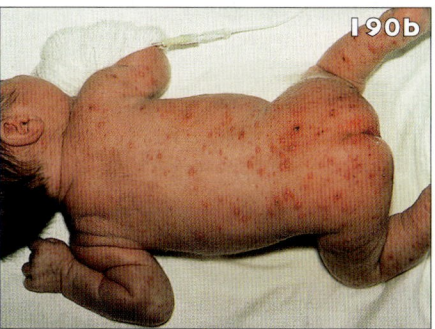

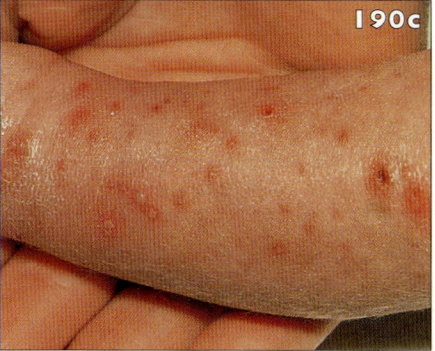

190 The mother shown developed severe chickenpox 2 days after delivery (**190a**). She brought her baby to the emergency department 3 days later with a fever and a rash (**190b, c**).
i. What are the characteristic features of the rash?
ii. Is the illness in the baby likely to be severe?
iii. What treatment is indicated?

191 A 4-year-old presents with a 24 hour history of pain in the hip. Examination shows 50% restriction of hip movements on the affected side apparently due to pain.
i. What is the most likely diagnosis?
ii. What is the important differential diagnosis?
iii. How do you distinguish between the above?

190 i. The rash characteristically starts on the trunk and spreads to the face, scalp, and proximal parts of the limbs. The initial lesions are macules, becoming papular and then vesicular within hours. The vesicles persist for 3–4 days, becoming pustular and finally crusted. The rash evolves by a series of crops so that lesions may be seen at all stages simultaneously.

ii. If the maternal rash appears less than 7 days before delivery or up to 2 days after delivery, the infant may receive a heavy inoculum of virus without maternal antibody. The infant is therefore at high risk of serious disseminated disease that can be fatal in up to 5% of cases. However, when the rash develops 3 days or more after delivery the risk is low.

iii. Acyclovir should be given. The baby should also receive varicella-zoster immunoglobulin.

191 i. The clinical signs suggest 'irritable hip' alternatively known as 'transient or toxic synovitis'.

ii. An urgent ultrasound showed an effusion on the right hip (**191**, large arrow). The image is essentially a sagittal 'cut' as if the hip were viewed from the side. Only the front of the joint is seen because the sound waves cannot pass through the bone. The dotted line demonstrates separation of the joint capsule from the femoral neck by ultrasonically 'dark' fluid. This is normal up to 2–3 mm (0.08–0.1 in) but here the gap is of the order of 7–8 mm (0.2–0.3 in).

iii. The most important differential diagnosis to consider is septic arthritis as the ultrasound does not differentiate the nature of the fluid. Septic arthritis is

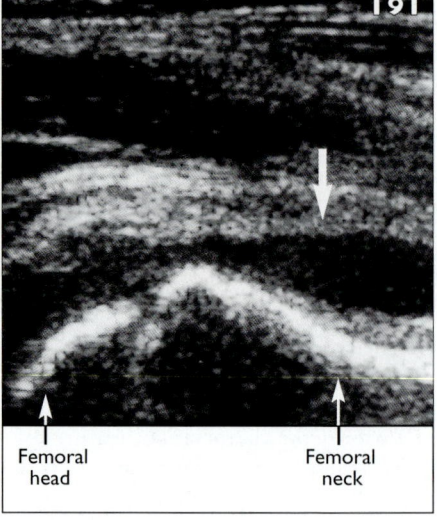

Femoral head

Femoral neck

unlikely clinically given that the child is otherwise well. An urgent full blood count and ESR will give confirmatory evidence. A throat swab is also taken as a streptococcal throat infection, clinical or subclinical is occasionally accompanied by an 'irritable hip'.

In some centers the radiologist will aspirate the effusion during the scan and send a specimen of the fluid for bacteriologic examination. Aspiration also has the effect of relieving discomfort.

192 How would you manage the patient in **191**?

193 A child was hit by a motor vehicle travelling at 35 mph (56 kph). The breath sounds are symmetrical but decreased. Heart sounds are in the correct position. The child has no jugular venous distension but has a prolonged capillary refill time of 5 seconds.
i. What does the X-ray show (**193**)?
ii. Could this be a tension pneumothorax?
iii. What other serious complications may be present?

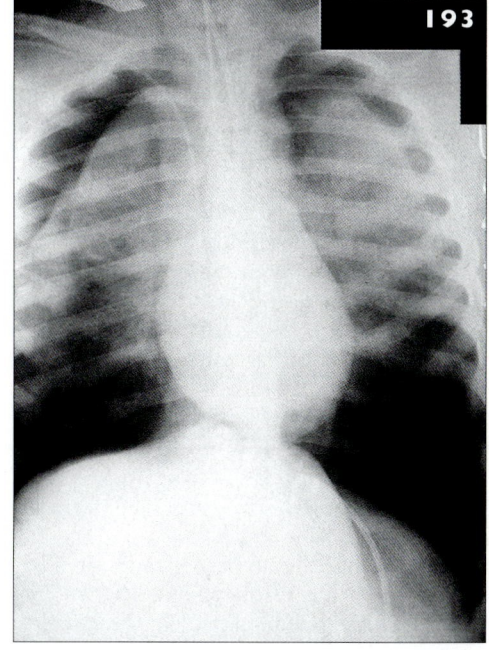

194 A case of traumatic commotio retinae is shown (**194**). Discuss the significance of the white area of the retina.

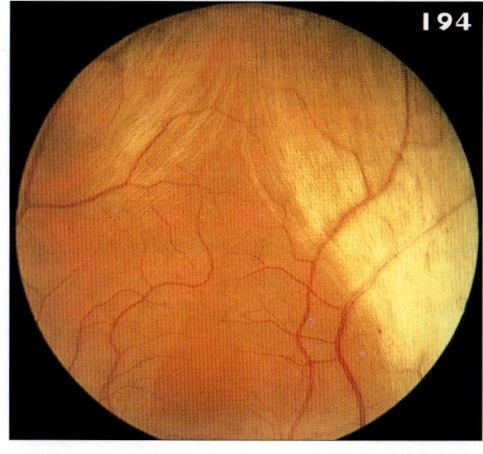

192 If the doctor is confident with the diagnosis of 'irritable hip' the child can go home for bedrest. It is advisable to review clinically in 2 days to check that the symptoms have at least improved before the child goes home for a full 10–12 days' rest. On review at 10–12 days, children with an effusion need a repeat ultrasound to ensure that the effusion has reduced or resolved. If there is no improvement clinically or on ultrasound then a 'frog lateral' X-ray is taken to check for other pathology, e.g. Perthe's disease. Sometimes early Perthe's disease will be seen but this short delay in diagnosis is unimportant. Rheumatological disorders seldom begin with an isolated synovitis.

If the signs and symptoms are severe enough to suggest infection the child requires admission for orthopedic assessment and observation even in the absence of a normal white blood cell count and ESR. Occasionally these are both normal in the very early stages of an osteomyelitis.

Occasionally children present with all the physical signs of irritable hip and despite normal investigations, including a normal ultrasound have a condition identical in both clinical signs and course to the classical irritable hip.

Despite the frequency of transient synovitis little is known about the cause of the condition and usually the parents are advised that it is due to a low grade viral infection (many parents will report that their child has recently had a cold or similar) or that the child probably 'overdid it' while playing and suffered a 'sprain' of the joint.

193 i. The chest X-ray shows bilateral pneumothoraces, compressed lungs, and possibly pulmonary contusions.
ii. This X-ray demonstrates bilateral tension pneumothoraces. The usual signs and symptoms of a tension pneumothorax include a shifted mediastinum, decreased breath sounds, asymmetric chest expansion, poor perfusion, and jugular venous distension. Several of these symptoms are absent because of the bilateral nature of the injury. Jugular venous distension was not seen secondary to hypovolemic status. This child improved significantly with the insertion of bilateral chest tubes.
iii. Other findings may include: pneumomediastinum, pneumopericardium, which if large may compromise cardiac function leading to hypotension, muffled heart sounds and cyanosis; subcutaneous emphysema; pneumoperitoneum; and other injuries to chest and abdomen.

194 The whitish color is an area of diffuse edema of the retina. This appears as a grayish sheen and the affected retina is not detached. Commotio may be localized or diffuse. If it involves the macula, the central vision is impaired to a variable extent. A repeat fundal examination with indirect fundoscopy is carried out 10–14 days later to ensure that no traumatic retinal tears or holes have formed.

If the media is opaque because of vitreous hemorrhages following trauma, observation is necessary to rule out an underlying retinal detachment or tear.

195 This infant developed fever, irritability and a rash over a period of 48 hours (**195**).

Describe the rash and provide a differential diagnosis for it. What is its cause and treatment?

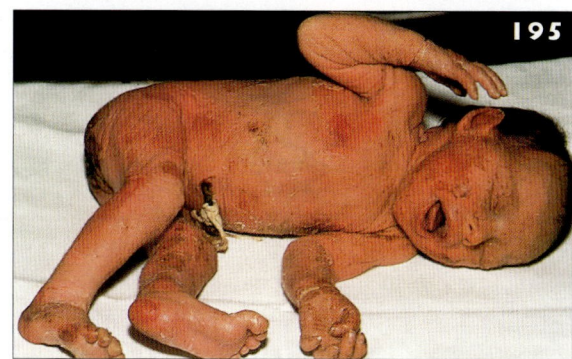

196 This 7-year-old child has fractured the mandible in the subcondylar region and through the opposite canine region (**196**). The left upper central incisor and both lower lateral incisors are intact but only partially erupted. The fracture is unstable. What problems may occur to the developing dentition and mandible?

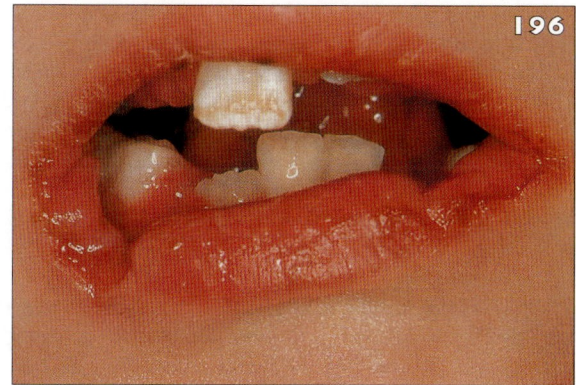

197 A mother brought her 4-year-old daughter in because she complained of itching and pain in her vaginal area (**197**). She is concerned about sexual abuse.
i. What is the diagnosis?
ii. What treatment do you recommend?

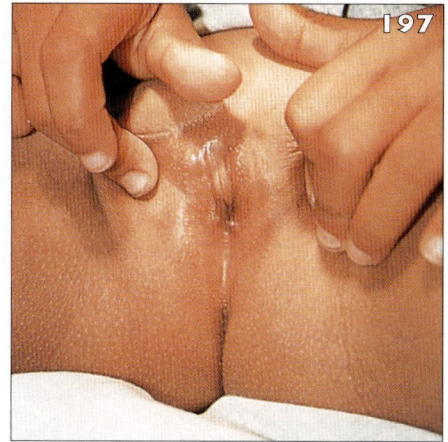

195 This infant has generalized erythema and areas of denuded skin with associated bullae. This is characteristic of 'scalded skin' syndrome, caused by epidermolytic toxin of *Staphylococcus aureus*. The differential diagnosis includes: bullous impetigo, sunburn, epidermolysis bullosa, drug induced epidermal necrolysis, and erythema multiforme.

Scalded skin syndrome starts with irritability, fever, erythema, and tenderness of the skin. The rash, which is caused by cleavage in the epidermal granular cell layer, starts in the skin folds before extending to the trunk and extensor surfaces. The Nikolsky sign (superficial skin layers rub off when the skin is gently rubbed) is present. Treatment of mild cases consists of oral flucloxacillin. In cases with systemic toxicity, the infant should be admitted to hospital for intravenous antibiotics and monitoring of fluids and electrolytes.

196 At 7 years of age the child is in the mixed dentition stage and both maxilla and mandible hold the developing adult dentition. The condyles have not yet reached their adult growth potential. The problems for the dentition at the fracture site is that eruption may be delayed or the developing tooth so damaged that its removal is indicated, either at the time of the fracture repair or at a later date. There may be present occlusal abnormalities in the developing dentition that require orthodontic realignment.

The condylar region of the mandible is a site of growth and if the growth center is disturbed unequal growth of the right and left mandibles may occur, resulting in deviation of the centerline and facial imbalance. The child requires regular review until growth stops to ensure this does not occur. If facial abnormalities result from the trauma, corrective orthognathic surgery will be required.

197 i. This girl has labial adhesions, a condition where the epithelium along the edges of the labia minora becomes traumatized by chronic irritation and adheres as it heals, with a translucent band along the line of adhesion. This process usually, although not in this case, involves the posterior part of the labia first and these are usually the first to adhere and the last to separate. The vulva thus appears flat and featureless as the clitoris, urethra, and hymen can be obscured. Cases of acquired adhesions occur most commonly in young girls between the ages of 3 months and 6 years. It has been postulated, but not proven, that such a condition may result from chronic irritation of sexual abuse. Abuse must therefore be considered but there is by no means indication for it in every case and as always, this diagnosis is most reliably made by a history taken from the child. Other presentations of labial adhesions include a discharge, dribbling of urine, and parental anxiety about a congenital abnormality.

ii. If the opening is large enough to allow adequate draining of vaginal secretions and urine, no therapy is necessary as the condition resolves with the estrogen effects occurring through puberty. If draining is a problem, estrogen cream twice daily and before bed is applied at the adhesion site. After separation, good hygiene must be practised and a diaper (nappy) ointment is applied at the site nightly for 6–12 months. Rarely, surgical excision is required. The partial obstruction to free flow of urine during micturition may predispose to urinary tract infection. It is useful to check such children for urinary tract infection.

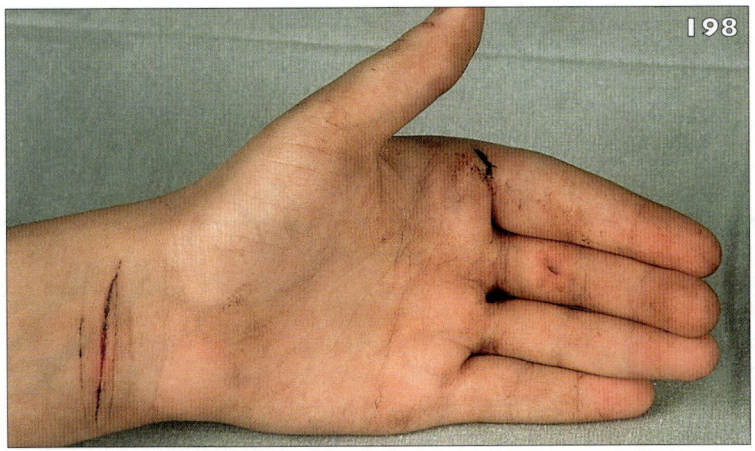

198 An adolescent girl was found unconscious at school by friends after threatening to 'kill herself'. Hand injuries are shown (**198**).
i. Which drugs are commonly associated with ingestions in adolescents?
ii. Describe the assessment you would undertake after acute treatment.

199 What abnormality do you see on this X-ray (**199a**)? What should the treatment be?

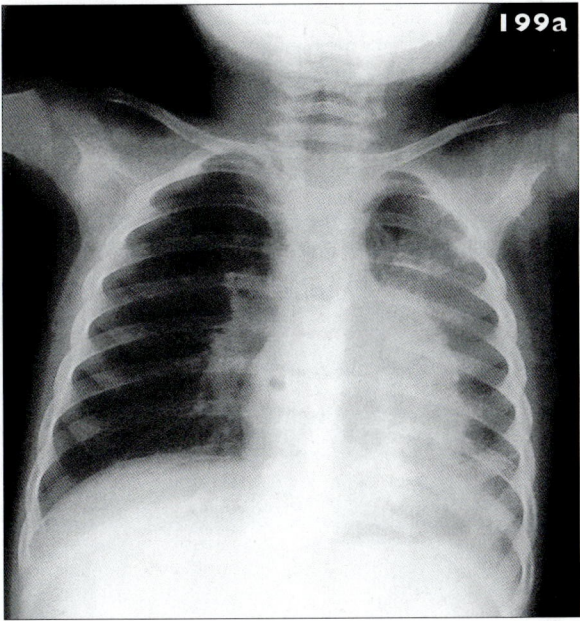

198 i. About 1 in 200 young people present to emergency departments with deliberate self harm, often in the form of an overdose. Many more do not present for acute medical care.

Drugs which are often taken in overdose include paracetamol (acetaminophen), benzodiazepines, tricyclic antidepressants, and other tranquillizers. Paracetamol levels must always be taken in the acute overdose because of the risk of acute hepatic necrosis if toxicity is missed. In addition, in this girl there are self-inflicted lacerations to her finger and wrist.

ii. Assessment of the young person is important in judging whether he or she is suicidal. Attention should be paid to: the actual harm incurred in the event, the degree of planning, suicidal intent ('Did you want to kill yourself?'), the perceived lethality of the event ('Did you think you would die?'), and the action taken by the young person after the event.

Assessment should also include the existence of associated psychiatric disorders (e.g. depression, eating disorder), and the presence of social and interpersonal difficulties in the young person's life. Child abuse sometimes predisposes to feelings of unworthiness. This should be sensitively explored. Patients with intent of self harm should be referred for psychiatric help.

199 The chest X-ray shows severe hyperinflation of the right lung with obstructive emphysema and displacement of the mediastinum to the left. The appearance is caused by partial obstruction of the right main bronchus and the most common cause of this in infancy is an inhaled foreign body.

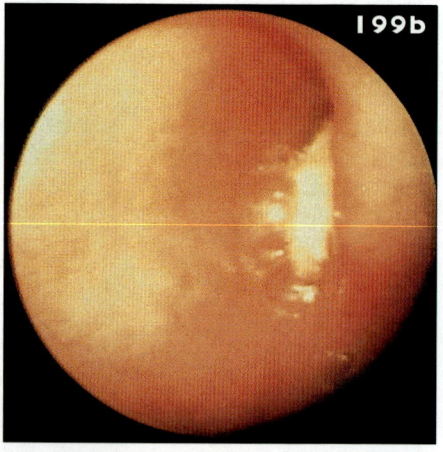

Such a case should be referred without delay for bronchoscopy and removal of the offending foreign body. The most common object found is a fragment of peanut, which should never be given to small children because of the oil contained in the peanut. There is a particularly severe reaction to such inhalation and if the foreign body is not removed, long term damage to the lung may follow. In this child a peanut could be seen in the bronchus on bronchoscopy (**199b**).

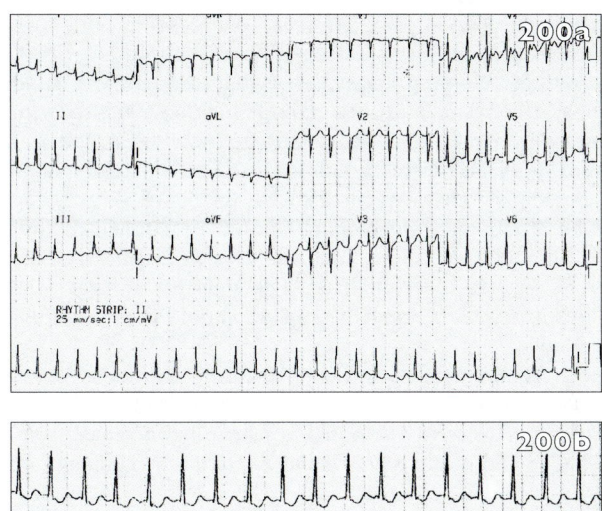

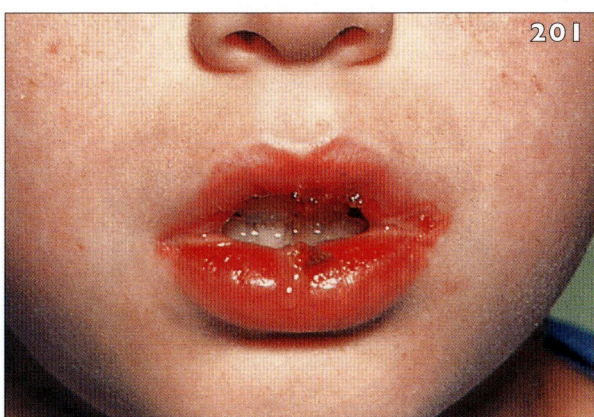

200 These ECG tracings of supraventricular tachycardia were obtained when a 4-year-old child presented to the emergency department with pallor, sweating, and feeling unwell for 12 hours (**200a, b**).
i. How do children with this condition commonly present?
ii. What treatment options are available?

201 This boy presented with a sore mouth and eyes 7 days after being treated with antibiotics by his primary care provider (**201**). What is the diagnosis and treatment?

200 i. Older children with supraventricular tachycardia who can describe their symptoms sometimes present with a history of a very rapid heart rate. However, the presentation in younger children varies. They may present with sudden episodes of pallor, restlessness or vomiting and their parents may have felt the rapid heart rate. A common presentation in infants is heart failure, the restless, lethargic baby having tachycardia, pallor, poor peripheral circulation, and an enlarged liver.

ii. If the child presents with tachycardia without heart failure, vagal stimulation should initially be attempted. An ice pack should be applied to the face so that it moulds the face for under 1 minute. One sided carotid sinus massage is difficult in infants but may be tried in older children. The Valsalva maneuver in older children can also revert this arrhythmia. Eyeball pressure should *not* be performed because of potential eye damage.

Pharmacological therapy consists of acute reversion with adenosine 0.05 mg/kg via very rapid intravenous injection. It has a very short half-life (only 10–20 seconds) so must be given quickly. This can be repeated in increasing increments of 0.05 mg/kg (i.e. 0.1 mg/kg, 0.15 mg/kg and so on) every 2 minutes until a maximum of 5 mg/kg has been given.

Of other drugs used in this condition, verapamil should not be used in infants under 1 year old because of the hypotensive side effects. Neostigmine should not be used in young infants.

If the patient is stable, digoxin in a loading dose of 15 µg/kg then 5 µg/kg 6 hours later will usually revert the supraventricular tachycardia over some hours.

In a patient who is in shock, synchronized cardioversion (1 joule/kg) should be initiated. This is uncommon in this age group.

201 The boy has sore ulcerated lips and mouth and sore eyes. He has Stevens–Johnson syndrome (erythema multiforme major).

This condition with bullae at mucocutaneous junctions is also associated with significant fluid losses from denuded skin, a reduced fluid intake, and pain.

The eye problems include a purulent conjunctivitis and uveitis and can be a rare cause of blindness.

Most of the children require admission to hospital for supportive therapy. The management is symptomatic and includes mouth washes, topical anesthetics, intravenous fluids if necessary, and antibiotics for secondary infection.

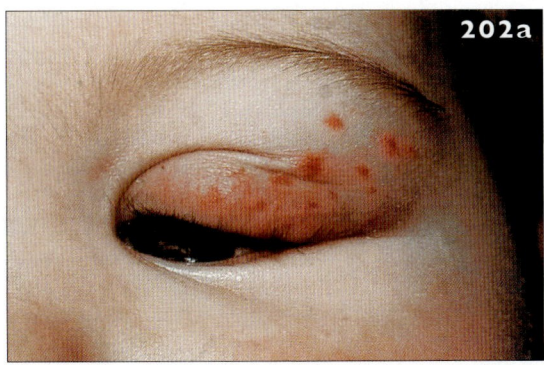

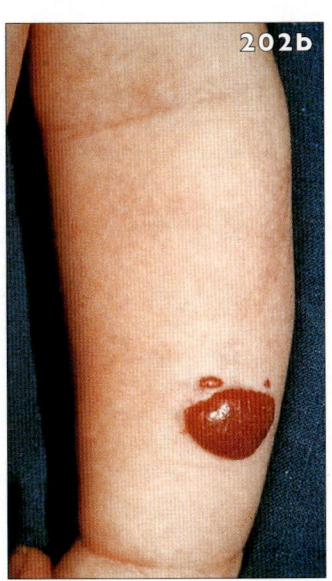

202 What is the significance of the hemangioma involving the eye which was noticed in a child presenting to the emergency department (202a)? This child also had a hemangioma of her arm (202b). What general advice can be given to parents of children with hemangiomas?

203 This child is seen in casualty with a 3 day history of wheezing. His mother says that he has mild asthma, for which he receives intermittent inhaled broncho-dilator treatment. He tends to be chesty a lot, and gets frequent courses of anti-biotics.

i. What clinical sign is shown (203)?
ii. What is the likely cause?
iii. How could you assess this further?
iv. What treatment would you give once he is over his acute problem?

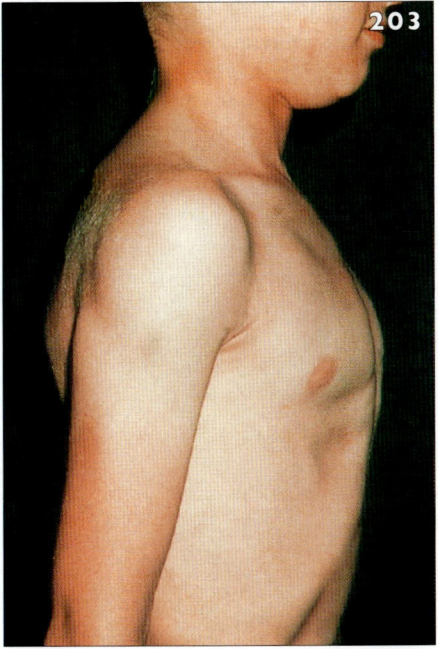

202 If the lesion is large then vision can be obstructed and lead to deprivation amblyopia. This can occur within weeks in some infants and so requires urgent referral to an ophthalmologist for assessment. Oral steroid therapy is indicated.

Hemangiomas which appear within the first week or two of life (not portwine stains or arteriovenous malformations) will usually resolve spontaneously over a variable period of years, after an initial period of proliferation. It is very uncommon to recommend surgery in the great majority of cases until resolution is complete, usually by age 8–10 years. It is suggested that 50% of hemangiomas resolve by the age of 5 years. Surgery can be carried out at this stage to excise redundant skin subcutaneous tissue that may be left.

Systemic steroid therapy is reserved for large lesions causing obstruction to vision, air passages, causing distortion of important structures such as facial features, or if giving rise to recurrent ulceration or bleeding.

Platelet trapping with very large lesions can lead to thrombocytopenia (Kasabach–Merritt syndrome) resulting in petechial hemorrhages or generalized purpura.

Any child on high dose steroid therapy for treatment of hemangiomas must not be immunized with vaccines containing live viruses.

Recently it has been recognized that proliferating hemangiomas in the very early stages can respond well to laser therapy.

203 i. The abnormality is a Harrison's sulcus, which is a concave deformity of the lower ribs anteriorly, due to the action of the diaphragm in the presence of decreased lung compliance.
ii. The commonest cause is poorly controlled asthma which reduces lung compliance by maintaining the lungs at the upper end of the pressure–volume curve.
iii. The lung function tests at the time of presentation will show an obstructive picture (reduced FEV_1, with less reduction in FVC), and there is likely to be more than 15% reversibility with salbutamol.

Poor asthma control may be demonstrable by twice daily peak flow monitoring for a few weeks.
iv. He needs to have regular inhaled preventive medication, which might be sodium cromoglycate or inhaled steroid.

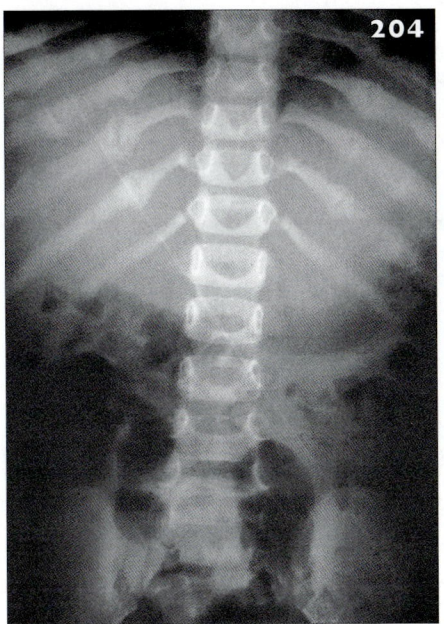

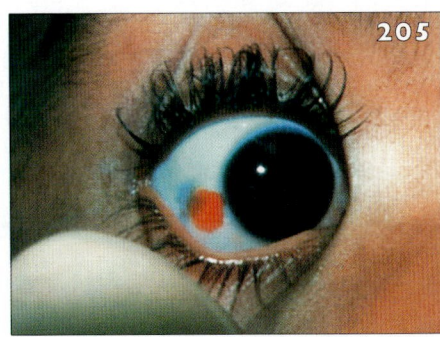

205 A battered child was brought to the emergency department for a medical examination before being placed in foster care. A subconjunctival hemorrhage was noted (205). What are the likely mechanisms of this injury?

204 An infant is brought into the emergency department with crying and abdominal distension. This X-ray of the abdomen is obtained (204). What diagnosis is confirmed?

206 This 3-year-old child presented with a history of runny nose and fever for 2 days followed by the appearance of a rash over the following 2 days (206). Her parents were concerned because some days later she vomited and was noticed to be staggering when attempting to walk. The family had just moved into an old house in the city. The child is on medication for repeated convulsions associated with fevers.
i. What is the likely cause of her unsteady gait?
ii. What investigations might be started in the emergency department?

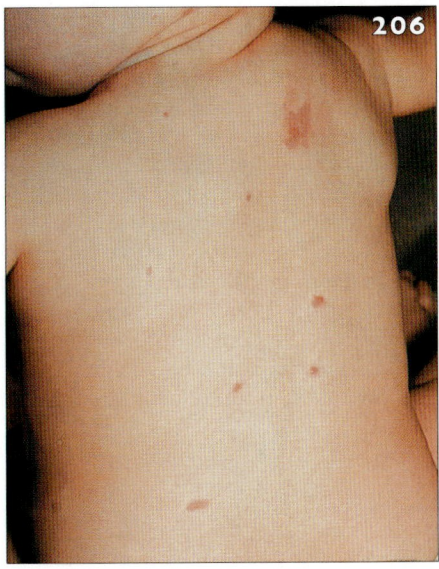

204 There are multiple healing rib fractures and there are also several acute injuries that are causing the baby to cry and to swallow air thus creating a large dilated gas bubble. Rib fractures are usually coincidental findings on X-ray taken for other conditions or as part of a skeletal survey in a child with other injuries. They are specific for nonaccidental injury provided that major trauma such as a motor vehicle accident, and bone diseases such as rickets, osteoporosis, or osteogenesis imperfecta have been excluded.

The fractures most commonly occur posteriorly, but also occur anteriorly and at the costochondral junction. The mechanism of injury is thought to be either by a blow to the chest or by squeezing the chest with the child held by the perpetrator with the thumbs anteriorly and the fingers pointing posteriorly causing compression of the rib cage. This is often found in association with intracranial injury after a child has been violently shaken.

This child would need a full pediatric assessment including X-ray skeletal survey to look for other bony injury. The child would need admitting to a safe place such as a pediatric ward while a full multiagency child protection investigation is undertaken.

205 Subconjunctival hemorrhages can be the result of either direct trauma to the eye or to hemodynamic forces transmitted to the eye during chest compression. They are common after vaginal delivery and may occur in association with severe coughing episodes. These hemorrhages are seen in a small percentage of abused children where they may be associated with retinal hemorrhages. Infants with subconjunctival hemorrhages should be examined by an ophthalmologist. Subconjunctival hemorrhages may also be associated with other ocular or facial injuries.

206 i. This child had prodromal fever and rhinorrhea with a rash which had macules, papules, and vesicles suggestive of chickenpox. Cerebellar ataxia may precede or follow the rash and the lack of signs other than cerebellar ones differentiate it from encephalitis or meningitis. Other infections associated with similar cerebellar findings include rubeola, mumps, rubella, echovirus infection, influenza, infectious mononucleosis, streptococcal infection, and salmonellosis.

Children with cerebellar ataxia can have a spectrum of signs from mild unsteadiness to truncal and limb ataxia, a reeling gait, an inability to sit unsupported or reach for objects, horizontal nystagmus, and slurred speech. There are no features of increased intracranial pressure nor any abnormal reflexes or sensory loss.
ii. In this particular child, other causes of the ataxia should be excluded. Simple tests which could be commenced in the emergency department include anticonvulsant levels, hemoglobin and blood film looking for the basophilic stippling of red cells in lead poisoning, urine test for proteins, and an X-ray of long bones looking for lead lines.

207 The child shown in **207** presented with a history of irritability for the previous few days.

i. What is the diagnosis and the differential diagnosis?

ii. At what age are hernias most often irreducible in children: 0–6 months, 1–6 years, 6–8 years?

iii. If you suspect an irreducible hernia to be present, what is the management?

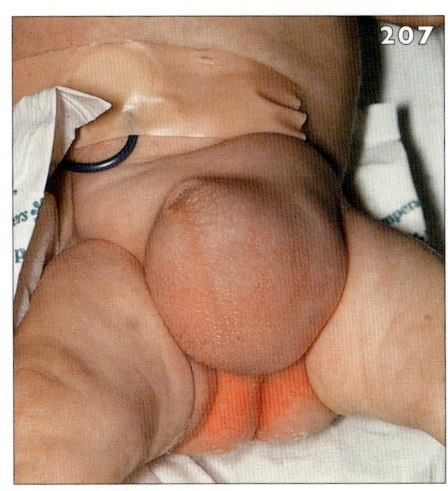

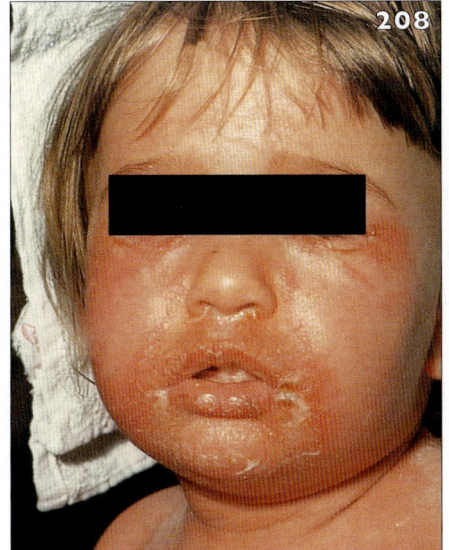

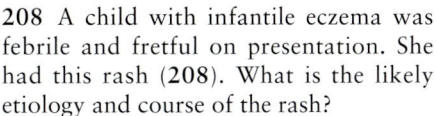

208 A child with infantile eczema was febrile and fretful on presentation. She had this rash (**208**). What is the likely etiology and course of the rash?

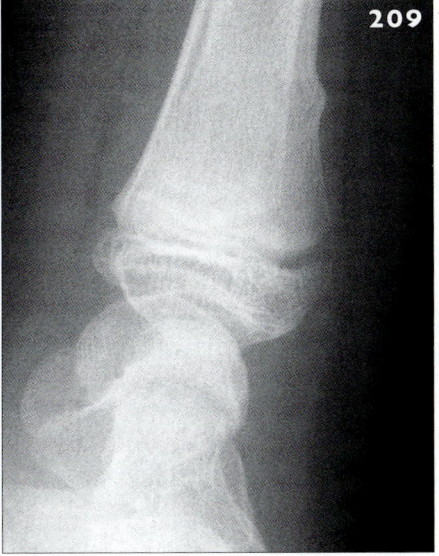

209 i. What is this injury of the distal radius called (**209**)?

ii. What are the mechanism and presenting features?

iii. What is the treatment and outcome?

207 i. The swelling in the right groin is an inguinal hernia, possibly incarcerated. In boys in this age group an irreducible hernia or torsion of the testis must be considered in the differential diagnosis.
ii. Hernias are most often irreducible in the 0–6 month age group.
iii. The patient should be referred to a pediatric surgeon for attempted reduction by taxis with morphine sedation if necessary. If this fails the child must be operated on without delay. The outlook for the testis is superior if the hernia can be manually reduced. If the hernia is incarcerated the testis is more vulnerable than the bowel.

208 She has an exfoliative eruption of scalded skin syndrome.

This is caused by an epidermolytic toxin produced by staphylococcus of phage type 2, 70/71 and 51. The site of infection is commonly the nose, throat, conjunctiva or deep wounds, and the umbilicus in neonates.

The staphylococcal toxin causes a macular rash of the face and flexures which gradually becomes generalized and tender. After 2 days flaccid bullae appear through high epidermal cleavage and the skin wrinkles and shears off. This exfoliation occurs especially in the groins, neck folds, and around the mouth. The epidermal shearing is superficial but the child should be admitted and fluid and electrolyte loss should be monitored. If large areas of skin are denuded, fluid replacement may be needed. The lesions dry, crust and desquamate leaving no sequelae.

This toxic condition is a medical emergency and the child should be treated promptly with antistaphylococcal antibiotics.

209 i. This is a buckle fracture (sometimes referred to as a torus fracture).
ii. These fractures are the result of a low energy compression injury which results in kinking of the relatively plastic bone of normal children. It usually occurs at the metaphysis.

These fractures sometimes only give relatively mild pain in young children and may present with some loss of use of the limb. It can be difficult to localize the injury in younger children as there is often no, or only minimal, pain on palpation of the limb and the child allows flexion and extension of the wrist but dislikes pronation and supination. It is usually easier to localize the pain in older children.
iii. The fracture is unicortical and almost never significantly angulated. It is a stable fracture which requires simple analgesia, a splint, and a sling. In most cases the splint can be discarded within 2 weeks. There are no long term problems.

Index

Index

Index

Index